Penguin Books
Drugs for All

Jenny Bryan is a freelance journalist who specializes in medical writing. She was brought up in Devon and took her degree in Biochemistry and Physiology at Queen Elizabeth College, London. Her first and last job was as science editor of the doctors' magazine *General Practitioner*, which she joined in 1976 and left in 1981. Since then she has written for a wide variety of newspapers and magazines including *The Times*, the *Guardian*, the *Sunday Express Magazine*, *New Scientist*, *Fitness* and *Successful Slimming*. She is currently medical correspondent to the *Sunday Telegraph*.

Much of her writing has centred on encouraging people to take more interest in their health and in making better use of medicines. She believes that it is time that much of the mystique surrounding the subject was done away with.

Jenny Bryan has won two awards for her articles which have enabled her to see the more remote parts of the world. Travelling – particularly to explore vanishing cultures and wildlife – is what she enjoys most, whenever time and money allow. In the absence of funds she reads, plays the piano, listens to music and occasionally plays tennis.

Jenny Bryan

DRUGS FOR ALL

based on the Central Television series

PENGUIN BOOKS

Penguin Books Ltd, Harmondsworth, Middlesex, England
Viking Penguin Inc., 40 West 23rd Street, New York, New York 10010, U.S.A.
Penguin Books Australia Ltd, Ringwood, Victoria, Australia
Penguin Books Canada Limited, 2801 John Street, Markham, Ontario, Canada L3R 1B4
Penguin Books (N.Z.) Ltd, 182–190 Wairau Road, Auckland 10, New Zealand

First published 1986

This book is based on the Central Independent Television series *Drugs for All?*
Television material copyright © Central Independent Television plc, 1986
Q   copyright © Central Independent Television plc, 1982

Made and printed in Great Britain by
Richard Clay (The Chaucer Press) Ltd, Bungay, Suffolk
Typeset in Times

For my brother, Chris

CONTENTS

ACKNOWLEDGEMENTS

I am grateful to everyone who gave so freely of their time to offer me help and advice during the writing of this book. But in particular I would like to thank Professor Michael Drury, Dr Conrad Harris, Dr Joe Collier, Jerry Shulman, Michael Cummings, Maddie Halliday, David Sharpe, Peter Llewelyn and David Taylor for their valuable comments on the many issues discussed in the book.

I would also like to thank International Computers Limited and Catherine Broadhead for their help in the preparation of the manuscript and Dr Chris Hawkey for reading it.

CHAPTER 1

What is a Drug?

In France they like suppositories; in the Middle East they put their faith in injections. Here in Britain we are less fussy; we consume over £1600 million worth of tablets, capsules, ointments and liquid medicines each year – and that does not include the £400 million worth of medicines we buy for ourselves at chemists and supermarkets.

What do we do with them all? A healthy proportion find their way into dustbins, down toilets or into the back of granny's medicine cabinet. But the vast majority are consumed with such fervour you would think they were the elixir of life.

If it seems as though we are a nation of pill-poppers, take a look at other Europeans and the Americans. While the average British citizen collects six or seven prescriptions from the doctor each year, across the Channel the French and Italians get ten and the traditionally stoic Germans take home an average of eleven prescriptions per year. But way ahead are the health-conscious Americans, who average between sixteen and seventeen prescriptions for each of the 200 million or so population.

If the type of prescription is anything to go by, the French and Italians are bothered most by their stomachs while here in Britain it is affairs of the heart and circulation which cause the most trouble. And if you always thought it was the Mediterranean types who tended towards histrionics you will be surprised to learn that the British are more likely to buy pain-killers than either the French or the Italians. Whatever happened to the days of 'grin and bear it' and a little suffering being good for the soul? It seems that nowadays we turn to the medicine cabinet at the first sneeze, tickly cough or pain in the head.

It is not as though drugs have brought us longevity, although more people are living into their seventies and eighties than ever before. But people who receive their telegram from the Queen are more likely to attribute their long lives to healthy living and a happy home than to the wonders of modern drugs.

In fact, drugs came on to the scene relatively late in terms of reducing death and serious illness. Better living conditions and improved standards of hygiene had reduced the annual death toll from 177 for every 10,000 population in 1900 to 125 for every 10,000 population in 1940, some five years before penicillin became generally available. Half a century later and the combined effects of antibiotics, vaccination and all the other advances in treatment of disease have contributed to a further fall to 117 deaths each year for every 10,000 population.

We may have increased the number of children reaching adolescence and beyond. But having overcome the big killer infections, we are left with the legacy of heart disease in middle and cancer in old age. And modern drugs as yet have had little impact on these harsh facts of life.

This is not to belittle the importance of modern drugs in improving the quality of life for countless millions of people with chronic diseases such as diabetes, arthritis and high blood pressure. The diseases are still there but, thanks to modern drugs, sufferers can live far more active and pleasurable lives than they would have done only thirty or forty years ago.

But there is a price to pay for every advance. And any drug which is strong enough to relieve symptoms or cure a disease is also strong enough to affect other parts of the body in a way which may be undesirable. A balance must be struck for any treatment and the benefits should outweigh the risks. The balance will vary; something which is worth suffering in the treatment of a severe disease may be far too unpleasant if the medicine is to be used to treat a trivial illness.

Drugs are not the only answer; an alternative form of treatment or a change in lifestyle may be a more effective solution but may still carry its own risk. Take the current controversy over exercise. People who run feel better, look better and frequently put the rest of us to shame. But occasionally they drop dead from the very condition they are running to avoid – a heart attack. Those are the unlucky ones and, on balance, the risk is small and in most cases worth taking.

Knowing the risks we run, whether in crossing the road, catching a plane, or backing the favourite for the Derby, we make our decision and accept the consequences. Should drug-taking be any different? We can hardly expect to understand our illness as well as our doctor. But surely we should take as much responsibility for our health and its upkeep as for our house, our car, our washing machine? We cannot diagnose the fault but we can consider the options for repair if they are explained to us.

There is a mystique about medicine which doctors sometimes seem intent on preserving. But, armed with the right questions and a willingness to understand the answers, we can get the information we need to help us make decisions about our drugs.

What do we need to know about our medicines in order to make more informed decisions about our treatment? Do we need those six prescriptions a year, not to mention the hoards of painkillers, indigestion tablets and cough mixtures we have got stashed away in our medicine cabinets? When does orthodox medicine let us down and what alternatives should we consider? No one has all the answers. But here are just a few.

How Drugs Work

Do you take drugs? Most of us would assume the question meant hard drugs like heroin. Most of us separate drugs into two categories. There are the addictive drugs with a capital 'D'; and there are the other sort, the ones we all take which make us feel better – the kind we believe we do not get hooked on.

The word drug encompasses far more than just the chemicals used by addicts and the medicines we take when we are ill. It actually means any substance which has an effect on the body. That sounds vague – and it is vague. It includes things we eat, things we drink, things we smoke, even things we breathe. But what most of us mean when we refer to drugs are the medicines we take to make us feel better when we are ill.

Some people prefer not to take medicines when they are ill; instead they have a hot toddy, a cup of herbal tea, a homeopathic remedy. But they are all drugs. They disturb the balance of chemicals constantly at work in the body and are therefore classified as drugs.

Remarkably little is known about the way in which many drugs actually work. It is enough that they are effective and do not appear to have too many unwanted side-effects. Most drugs fall into one of two categories; either they boost supplies of chemicals in the body which are too low or they suppress levels of chemicals or block their effects when they are out of control or have risen too high for our own good. Additionally, there are drugs such as vaccines which are designed to make the body produce chemicals it would not normally make except under attack.

In general, though, more of the drugs we take are geared to suppressing rather than boosting chemicals in the body. Tranquillizers, for example, are thought to dampen supplies of chemicals which make us nervous. An important group of heart drugs, the beta-blockers, stop the heart from overreacting to the chemicals which make it jumpy. And the anti-arthritic drugs stop pain-causing chemicals from being made.

In these cases, the medicine competes with the natural chemical for its place in the tissues. Each natural chemical has its own special slot on or inside cells through which it passes messages in order to be effective. Many drugs are designed to cause a sort of 'crossed line'. They are roughly the same size and shape as the body's own chemicals so they are able to get into the same slots and prevent signals from getting through.

Drugs which boost supplies of chemicals in diabetes, for example, also latch on to these empty slots in the tissues. But because the drug is mimicking the body's own natural chemical it gives a power surge to the system, instead of a crossed line.

Ideally, drug manufacturers would like to design new medicines to interact precisely with recognized slots – or 'receptors' to give them their scientific name – in the tissues. But frequently they find out how a drug works long after it has been put on to the market. An educated guess starts them on the trail of a drug which might work and it is only much later that they find out just why it does.

For centuries, herbalists were able to treat and cure a wide variety of illnesses by crushing a motley collection of roots and leaves which had been found to have medicinal properties. For most of this century, doctors and drug companies have tried to make medicines in the laboratory out of synthetic chemicals, and thus maintain more control over the quality and quantities of their products.

But in the last five to ten years there has been a shift back towards natural medicines. Recognizing that they have been ignoring hundreds, and perhaps thousands, of plant chemicals, many companies have embarked on research programmes into natural products. In particular, many third-world countries are concentrating on developing their drugs from plants because synthetic drugs have become so expensive.

How a drug works in the body is not the only thing which determines whether we feel better. Other factors, not least whether we have faith in our medicine, affect how well it works. Nowhere is this better demonstrated than in the use of so-called 'dummy pills' or placebos.

All in the Mind?

The word 'placebo' is Latin and means 'I shall please'. In medicine it refers to a form of treatment which is not actually expected to do any good. Curiously, it sometimes does a lot of good and is frequently very pleasing to the patient.

A delightful story told recently in one of the medical journals referred to a woman whose blood pressure was exceedingly pleased with a placebo. She had been entered into a major Medical Research Council study to find out whether treating slightly raised blood pressure can prevent heart attacks. Her blood pressure was slightly up so she was put on a course of treatment which turned out to be the placebo rather than the active therapy. Drugs are frequently compared with placebos in trials in order to find out whether the drug has more effect than chance in improving the patient's condition.

Unknown to herself or her doctor the woman took the placebo for the five years of the trial and her blood pressure went down satisfactorily. At the end of the study the doctors decided she could stop taking the placebo. But within a few weeks her blood pressure went up and she needed treatment. This time she was given a real drug – after all, you do not treat a disease like high blood pressure with a placebo, do you? No one knows why placebos work. But they do, sometimes in as many as one in three people to whom they are given.

The confidence we place in our medicine can have a significant effect on how well it works. We stand a far better chance of recovering from an illness if we believe the medicine will work than if we have no faith in it. Why else would we believe the claims of some pain-killers to bring instant relief when we know that it *must* take fifteen to twenty minutes for the drug to be absorbed by the body and relieve the pain?

How often have you said, 'I feel much better', when asked if your headache has gone only a few minutes after taking a pain-killer? You expect to feel better . . . and so you do. That does not mean you did not have a headache in the first place, just that in swallowing a pill you somehow mobilized your own natural pain-control mechanisms to relieve the headache before the drug had time to get there. The body's natural pain-killers are being credited with many of our mechanisms for overcoming our ills, from enabling eastern mystics to walk across hot coals to putting a smile on joggers' faces and making them feel well when the rest of us know they are going through torture. It may be that this ubiquitous breed of brain chemicals also has some part to play in placebo responses.

It is not just faith in medicine which can make it work; faith by proxy, through our doctor, can do just as well. Each time a general practitioner (GP) hands a patient a prescription with the reassuring words, 'I'm sure this will clear it up', the potency of the medicine is increased in some way.

The size, shape and colour of a drug can also affect whether it works. People are very wary of changes in the appearance of tried and trusted medicines. If they are used to little pink tablets for their heart they do not like large white ones to be substituted.

It is no coincidence that manufacturers have given strong bold colours to drugs to combat degenerative diseases such as arthritis and circulatory illnesses, nor that many of the tranquillizers come in gentle pastels. A study carried out in the Seventies showed that red placebos were far more effective pain relievers for arthritis sufferers than blue or green, and yellow was not worth trying. Drug companies go to considerable trouble to ensure they are promoting the right image for their drug, from its size, shape and colour, to its packaging and promotion.

The fact that so many outside factors can influence how well medicines work is interesting to both patients and scientists. But should the doctor play on these factors when we go to the surgery or should he take the time to explain that our illness is short and self-limiting, that we do not need drugs and that we should simply wait for our symptoms to clear up? How many of us would accept such a message, which is in effect telling us that we are making a fuss and should not really be in the doctor's surgery.

Basically, the doctor can take one of two approaches to the patient who comes into surgery with a mixture of apparently unrelated, minor symptoms. The first is to listen to the symptoms, decide that they are not serious but hand out a prescription for an innocuous drug to ensure that the patient leaves the surgery satisfied. Convinced that he is in fact 'ill', he goes off to collect his drugs and will bear his illness with fortitude until it is cleared up by his drugs.

The alternative and more difficult approach for both doctor and patient, is for the doctor to listen to the symptoms sympathetically but tell the patient she is not sure how they relate to one another and that she believes that whatever illness the patient is suffering will be short-lived and will pass without any medication. To this the patient can respond in one of two ways. Either he will glare at the doctor for not taking him seriously. How dare she suggest that he is malingering? Or he can breathe a sigh of relief that there is nothing much wrong and be glad that his body can get over whatever is ailing it without the need for drugs.

Of course, the doctor must be sure that there is no underlying worry which is showing itself in apparently unrelated symptoms. And she must be sure that, in not giving a prescription, she is not undermining the patient's confidence to such a degree that he will not return when there is something seriously wrong.

For example, the lonely old lady whose dog has just died and who comes to the surgery for a chat and a 'pick-me-up' may well need a prescription to ensure that she comes back again and does not sit uncaring of herself at home until hypothermia, malnutrition or neglect speed her into permanent care or even death.

It is a fine line to travel, distinguishing between those few who really do need a placebo and those who do not. Some of us might feel insulted that we are being given a drug which the doctor does not think we need and has no expectation of it having any effect. We would be quite irate if a garage mechanic changed a perfectly healthy clutch or recommended a new radiator for our car when the old one was not leaking. So why are we so much more happy to over-treat our bodies?

When we are paying the bills directly we try to get away with minimum servicing or repair charges. But when the bill is not in front of us in black and white all our instinctive desire for a bargain seems to disappear. If the National Health Service's (NHS) drugs bill goes up we will have to pay more in taxes to compensate. Or other areas of the health service will be cut back to pay the extra costs.

So it may be worthwhile waiting a few days before you go to the doctor; your aches and pains may go away on their own – though if you are really worried never hesitate to go in search of help. And when the doctor says your illness will clear up and you do not need a prescription, feel glad that she is not fobbing you off with a placebo.

Tablet, Injection or Suppository?

Medicines come in all shapes, sizes, colours and forms. The ultimate goal of any medicine is its site of action. It is not doing much good in your mouth, stomach or even bloodstream; it is only working when it is slotted into those sites on the tissue where it blocks or boosts the body's own chemicals.

Actually monitoring a drug latching on to receptors and dropping off again is a highly skilled job. So drug levels – and potential effectiveness – tend to be monitored in the blood. Once in the blood there is a fair chance that most of the drug will reach its site of action; so doctors measure effectiveness by how quickly a drug gets into the blood and how long it stays there.

The quickest way of getting a drug into the blood is by injection or infusion; in emergencies this is how it is done. In some cases injections are needed because the drug would be broken down and made useless by enzymes in the stomach if it was taken by mouth. Insulin is one such drug.

Drugs designed to work on the skin are usually given in ointment form since they will get to their target site more quickly that way. And drugs for the bottom end of the bowel or the genital tract are often given in suppository or pessary form so that they do not have to go through the blood to reach where they are needed.

Ever since an Egyptian medicine man popped a foul-tasting pill down a patient's throat nearly 3500 years ago, people have been looking for ways of making medicines work more quickly and controlling how long they go on working.

We take it for granted that any tablet we swallow will dissolve somewhere between mouth and intestine, make its way into the bloodstream, and then take the fastest possible route to the trouble spot and make it better. But it was not always so. Before the Norman Conquest, physicians were making pills look very pretty – wrapping them in silver or gold – but rarely did they release their contents or have any effect. Either they disintegrated before they made it to the mouth or they failed to dissolve and were next seen gracing the medieval chamber-pot.

It was not until 1834 that French pharmacists invented the gelatin capsule which dissolved in the stomach and ensured that the drug it contained stood a better than even chance of getting into the blood. Alongside this came the development of the compressed tablet which was the forerunner of today's drugs.

In the last forty years research has concentrated on finding ways of controlling how a drug is released from its outer coating – be it a tablet, capsule, suppository or injection. Just how quickly the drug needs to be released depends on the nature of the illness being treated.

In the case of a headache or indigestion, the chosen drug needs to get to the pain as quickly as possible and unload all its power for instant relief. Even so, it takes a minimum of twenty minutes for such a drug to get to the stomach and intestine, dissolve, get itself transported across the wall of the gut and into the blood.

In a chronic condition, a totally different type of response is required. Take high blood pressure, for example. A fast-acting drug is needed but the drop in blood pressure must not be too sudden and the drug must continue working for many hours; the same goes for the treatment of inflammation in someone with arthritis. To some extent the duration of action of a drug will depend on the nature of the drug itself. Some drugs are naturally excreted more quickly than others. But the process of getting the drug to work and making it go on working can also be affected by the nature of its packaging – how the tablet or capsule is put together.

The simplest way of doing this is to coat granules of drug in materials of different thickness. These are then compressed into a tablet or capsule. The granules with the thinnest coating dissolve first and those with the thickest coating dissolve last, thus ensuring a continual release of drug over many hours. A newer method of achieving the same end is to wrap the drug in a sponge-like gel. When this hydrogel comes into contact with watery body fluids it swells up and allows the water to get into the spongy compartments containing the drug. The drug dissolves and flows slowly out of the tablet and into the body.

A similar system of allowing water to pass in at a controlled rate and dissolve crystals of drug wrapped in their own mini-capsules has been used to great effect in many drugs, such as anti-arthritic and antibiotic agents. Each dose of the drug can contain hundreds of thousands of these tiny capsules and the rate at which they release their contents can be controlled by the nature of the material used to clothe them.

A refinement of this method has used a sort of chemical pump to push the drug out of the tablet. The system works like a bellows, with water entering the lower compartment of the tablet and building up pressure in the top compartment to push the drug out through a tiny hole. This can be achieved in a tablet only the size of a fingernail.

In each case, the rate at which the drug is released is carefully controlled. Before such methods were devised the drug was released in one large lump within an hour or two of swallowing it. Initially, a large amount of drug would be present in the blood and then levels would begin to tail off to ineffective levels long before the next dose of drug was due, perhaps eight hours later. The only alternative was to take frequent small amounts of drug. But anyone who has had to take two or more different types of drugs three or four times a day knows how difficult it can be to remember to take their drugs at the right time.

The rate at which the drug is released can also be affected by a number of other factors – whether it is taken on an empty or a full stomach, whether you eat a fatty or high-carbohydrate diet and what other drugs you are taking at the same time.

The importance of precisely controlling insulin levels in diabetics is reflected in the development of a special pump implanted under the skin of a diabetic which releases insulin at a carefully controlled speed. The simplest of these devices releases insulin to coincide with meals but the most sophisticated devices can actually sense when blood-sugar levels are getting high or low and adapt the insulin infusion accordingly.

However, most diabetics can keep their blood-sugar levels under control quite easily with regular injections of insulin. Pumps implanted under the skin have been used to great effect to treat other conditions. One is infertility, when the dose of hormone must exactly mimic the body's own natural production. Pumps can ensure this happens and improve the chances of a pregnancy. The pump system is a variation of the well-established practice of infusing drugs directly into the bed-bound patient to ensure that levels of the drug are maintained. This is especially important with drugs which are metabolized very quickly by the body. Both infusions and pump systems are useful in controlling severe and chronic pain, such as occurs in cancer patients and people who have undergone major surgery and are in pain for days or weeks after their operation. It is no good keeping to a rigorous time-schedule for handing out drugs to such patients. Some cancer victims treated in general hospitals can still find themselves being told to wait another two hours for their next dose of pain-killing drugs. But the more enlightened approach taken by specialized clinics is that the patient should never be in pain and that drugs should be taken before and not after the pain breaks through; hence they aim to ensure that a constant level of the drug is maintained in the bloodstream.

The needle is not the only alternative when a drug is either destroyed in the stomach or fails to dissolve. One of the newest techniques for ensuring that the drug gets to its target is to incorporate it in a plaster and stick it on the skin.

We are all used to rubbing ointments into the skin for spots and rashes, but the idea of curing chest pain through the skin may come as rather a surprise. For years, a drug called glyceryl trinitrate was used to relieve sudden bouts of chest pain caused by blockage in the arteries to the heart – angina. But, like its explosive counterpart, TNT, the drug tended to be rather unstable. To avoid it being metabolized in the liver before it could work, glyceryl trinitrate was used to relieve acute attacks by placing a lozenge under the tongue and allowing it to dissolve. The advent of the concept of giving drugs across the skin gave the drug a new lease of life.

The sticking-plaster which contains the drug has five layers. Nearest to the skin is a layer of adhesive which sticks the plaster to the skin. A thin membrane separates the reservoir containing the drug from the adhesive layer. The membrane is the crucial part since it controls the speed at which the drug seeps from this container and into the skin. A protective backing on the outside of the plaster gives it the same appearance as any ordinary sticking-plaster and prevents leakage of the drug.

In theory this sort of system could be used for a number of other drugs. But its effectiveness depends on how easily the drug permeates the outer layers of the skin and finds its way to the blood capillaries which are in the lower layers of the skin and carry the drug to the main blood system. If a drug is already effective taken orally or in some other satisfactory formulation then there is no need to go to the time and expense of devising a skin system of release. One other drug has been incorporated into skin patches and is used to prevent severe travel sickness. This drug, hyoscine, causes an alarming increase in heartbeat when given by mouth but the skin system avoids this and other side-effects.

Most slow-release preparations – from the microcapsules within a capsule to the skin-patch system – are designed to release their contents slowly over periods from eight to twenty-four hours. The subcutaneous pumps generally contain sufficient supplies of drug for several weeks or months. But it is also possible to extend the release period to three or four months by implanting pellets of drug wrapped in thick gel which allows the drug to permeate out only very slowly.

These 'depot' injections have been used for both contraception and for hormone-replacement therapy for women experiencing the menopause. Once implanted they cannot be removed and if the patient is unfortunate enough to experience side-effects as can occur with the contraceptive injections, she must simply wait three to four months for the effect to wear off. The skin has not been the only target for implants. Tiny implants have been used to release drugs into the eye and radioactive implants have been used to destroy cancerous tissue particularly in inaccessible areas such as the brain.

In addition to controlling the release of drugs, researchers have also been trying to devise methods of targeting drugs – making them 'home into' the precise areas where they are needed. For example, cancer drugs are geared to kill cells; unfortunately they are not particularly discriminating about which cells they kill – healthy or diseased. This is why enormous effort is going into making drugs more specific to the receptors to which they become attached on the tissues. Scientists are trying to provide them with a sort of rudder to control the direction in which they go. They can attach chemicals to the drugs which will only lock on to certain types of tissue and prevent them from getting diverted into cells where they are not wanted.

The same principles, applied to other drugs, could reduce their likelihood of causing side-effects. For example, the beta-blockers which are used to reduce blood pressure compete with natural nerve transmitters which lock into the beta-receptors of the heart and circulatory system. Unfortunately this type of receptor is also present in the lungs. Normally, this does not matter. Most people can cope with having receptors in their heart and blood vessels. But for asthmatics, whose lung passages are in poor condition, the effect can be catastrophic. Blocking the receptors in their lungs can cause a narrowing of the tubes and bring on a serious asthmatic attack. For this reason, beta-blockers cannot be used to treat high blood pressure or heart-beat abnormalities in asthmatic patients. There are other drugs which can be used but the beta-blockers – a very useful group of drugs – are out.

If in future scientists can develop something which will distinguish the beta-receptors in the heart from those in the lungs and attach it to the drugs as a sort of signpost, they can avoid the drugs having an effect on the lungs and open up a new area of treatment of high blood pressure for people who also suffer from asthma.

Merely coming up with a new drug is not the whole process. A drug company must decide not only the ideal dose or range of doses for different patients, but must also decide on the formulation. Will the drug be most effective as tablet, capsule, injection, suppository, skin preparation or infusion? What can be done to make it home in specifically on the area where it is most needed? And how can its activity be maintained at a constant level throughout the day?

CHAPTER 2

What Do We Expect from Our Drugs?

'I expect them to work, of course.'

'I wish there was something which really worked, without all these side-effects.'

'The orange ones; they do the trick.'

'They worked last time so I expect they'll clear it up this time too.'

'These are for my wife to clear up an infection she got as a result of taking some other drugs.'

'I don't know much about them at all.'

'Oh, I don't take drugs. I have these homeopathics.'

We have all come to expect a great deal from the drugs we take. Newspapers and magazines report new wonder drugs and breakthroughs and advertisements promise us instant relief. Yet only a very small proportion of drugs on the market were actually designed to cure disease. Most drugs are designed to relieve symptoms – to make us feel better without necessarily getting to the root of the illness or correcting the fault.

No cold remedy cures a cold. An aspirin will reduce a temperature and relieve a headache. A nasal decongestant may unblock a stuffy nose. And a cough mixture may soothe a tickly throat. But the cold goes on until the body wins its fight with the cold virus. The same is true for many other drugs, both those prescribed by a doctor and those bought at a chemist. Someone with diabetes is given insulin because he cannot make sufficient hormones for himself. Stop the insulin and he will not start producing his own. Someone who suffers from high blood pressure can be given drugs to reduce it. He will feel better but the disease is not cured. Whatever caused his blood pressure to rise in the first place will not go away and if treatment is stopped, his blood pressure will generally go up again. The asthmatic child whose wheezes disappear completely when given drugs to dilate the tubes in his lungs still remains an asthmatic; stop the drug and the wheezes will return.

Some drugs do cure an illness. Antibiotics can kill life-threatening bacteria in serious infections. Certain types of cancer – sadly, only a small minority – can be cured with drugs. In some cases drugs can be used to tide a patient over while the body puts itself right. Used correctly, tranquillizers and sleeping pills can bring relief in the short term while body and soul put themselves in order. Antidepressants do not have to mean treatment for life. Doses can gradually be reduced until sufferers find that they no longer need treatment.

It is often difficult to distinguish how much a drug has contributed to the improvement of a patient's condition and how much is simply the natural course of the disease – good patches and bad. But we should be aware of the purpose of our treatment – whether it is to be a short course for immediate cure or relief of symptoms, or whether it will be a long-term therapy, perhaps for life, with or without the possibility of cure.

Understanding Our Drugs

An average consultation with the doctor lasts five minutes. Two out of three patients leave the surgery with a prescription and an indeterminate number of people hooked into the 'repeat-prescription' system get their drugs without even seeing a doctor. But how many of us really need the drugs we are prescribed and do we know enough to get the most out of them?

Studies have shown that we forget nearly half of what we are told in the surgery. And the more we are told, the more we forget. Someone told two things by the doctor will remember both, someone told four things will forget one, and someone told eight things will forget half. In general, we tend to remember what we are told first, but doctors frequently leave information about how to take our drugs until last. So we may come away with our heads full of relatively unimportant information.

Intelligence and age are surprisingly unrelated to how much we remember but one of the most important factors which will impede our memory is anxiety. And unfortunately, going to the doctor can be traumatic for a lot of people.

A quick examination, a glance at his notes and the average patient is out of the doctor's door with a prescription before he has had a chance to ask what the tablets are and how to take them. Hoping that the label on the medicine will remind him of what the doctor said he takes it out of the bag in the chemist's shop only to find the immortal words 'take as directed' or 'as before' on the label.

The answer may be some form of written reminder of the information given verbally by the doctor when he sees you. A few doctors already produce their own hand-written or typed advice sheets. So it can be worth asking. Alternatively, many doctors are quite prepared to write down briefly what they have said. In which case, what exactly do we need to know?

It is not always possible for a GP to diagnose what is wrong, particularly if she needs the results of tests before making a diagnosis. But in the majority of cases she can probably hazard a guess at an infection, a strained muscle, or a digestive problem, for example. So first of all find out what the doctor thinks is wrong and make sure you know what the answer actually means! Doctors over-use scientific terms, so while diverticulosis or dysmenorrhoea may sound impressive they do not convey a lot. So make your doctor use words of one syllable!

The name of the drug she is going to prescribe is probably less important than what it is going to do. Drug names tend to be long and difficult to pronounce. It probably is not then worth asking the exact drug name in the surgery but make sure the name of the drug is on the bottle from the pharmacy and try to memorize it later.

When you leave the surgery you should know what the drug is going to do and, most important of all, how much and when to take it. Be sure that you know:

– how many tablets you should be taking,
– whether you should be taking them at any particular time of the day,
– how long you should go on taking them for.

Most drugs get into the bloodstream quickest when the stomach is empty – they do not have to compete with food for a passage through the intestine. But some drugs – common pain-killers such as aspirin and many anti-arthritic drugs – should not be taken on an empty stomach because they may cause irritation to the stomach and intestine.

Mealtimes are often a good reminder for taking drugs. If you are told to take a drug three or four times a day it is best to space them as equally as possible but it is rarely necessary to get up in the middle of the night to take drugs. The exceptions are antibiotics which generally have to be taken at accurately timed intervals, so that bacteria do not have a chance to reassert themselves while drug levels are low during the night. But, in general, one tablet at breakfast, one at about lunchtime, one at supper and one before bed will probably suffice. If you are taking two or more drugs try to space them so that you can take them at the same time. It is unlikely that you would have been given drugs which do not mix and by cutting down the number of times a day you have to take medicines you reduce the risk of forgetting.

If you are taking sleeping pills be sure not to take them with too long a gap before you get into bed. But do not wait until you get into bed or it will be twenty minutes before they start working. Ideally, they should be taken fifteen to twenty minutes before bedtime, perhaps with a milky drink. There is nothing worse than waking up cold and stiff in an armchair in the early hours of the morning because you got hooked on the late movie after taking your sleeping pill.

A few drugs, such as some contraceptive pills, have to be taken at the same time each day. (This is not so important with the combined hormone pills although it is good to get into a routine of taking the Pill either last thing at night or when you wake up.) But if you are on one of the Pills containing only progestogen it is very important that you take the Pill at the same time each day or you risk bleeding or pregnancy.

In a few cases some foods should be avoided when taking drugs. Some antidepressant drugs fall into this category and patients should not eat foods containing a chemical called tyramine found, for example, in cheese and in red wine. Patients on these drugs should be given a list of foods to avoid.

Drugs should never be washed down with alcohol but few people on long-term therapy cannot have the occasional drink. In general, people taking tranquillizers or antidepressant drugs should not drink but doctors may feel that the occasional glass of sherry will not hurt.

Having established what we are taking drugs for and when not to take them, most of us want to know how quickly we will start to feel better. Some drugs start to take effect immediately but others have to accumulate in the body to achieve their maximum effectiveness. Antidepressants are a good example of the latter.

It will take two or three weeks to build up enough of these drugs in the blood for patients to begin to feel better. But, unless they are told that they will have to wait a while to feel better, many people get discouraged because the drugs do not seem to be working, and may stop taking the drugs before they have had a chance to do their job.

It is important to complete the course of tablets you are given with some drugs. Although most of us know how important it is to take a whole course of antibiotics, it is very tempting to stop after two or three days when we feel better. But at that stage of the infection, there may well be a few bacteria left alive, which without the antibiotics to finish them off will come back. The same applies to drugs taken as pessaries for infections such as thrush. Although all signs and symptoms of the infection may have disappeared after two days' treatment, every pessary must be used or you could find yourself back at square one the very next week and the organism, having had a taste of the medicine, will be much better able to resist the drugs the next time around.

The last piece of information you should get straight before you leave the surgery concerns whether you are likely to suffer any unwanted side-effects with your medicine. In some cases these may be part and parcel of the treatment – in fact its effectiveness may depend on these effects. In other cases the problems are less common but none the less occur sufficiently frequently for you to be aware that they could happen to you.

A good example of a group of drugs which fall into the first category are diuretics. These drugs are given to lower blood pressure and they do this by increasing the amount of water passed as urine. There can be quite a substantial increase in the number of times you will need to go to the toilet and this can be very embarrassing if you are not expecting it. Elderly people in particular can be deeply embarrassed and have their confidence shaken if they are not aware that this might happen. And those who are confined to bed should have a commode or bedpan to hand at all times until they know how often they will need to go. It is very easy to label the old and infirm incontinent without taking account of the effects of their drugs.

When it comes to drugs with less obvious effects, doctors are constantly faced with the question of how much they should warn their patients of possible side-effects. The powers of suggestion are very strong and it is all too easy to start feeling sick, tired or lethargic because these are known possible side-effects of our drugs.

On the other hand, it is unfair to let people battle against a lethargy they can do nothing about because they are not aware it is caused by their drugs. Often patients work out for themselves that they are experiencing side-effects from their medicine. But they may be so worried that they stop taking it. All that may be needed is a few simple words of warning and reassurance from the doctor when the drugs are prescribed.

The best thing is for a doctor to warn patients of the most common and probably quite minor side-effects of a drug. And she can advise patients to come back and see her if they are worried about side-effects, rather than suddenly stopping the medicine altogether. In some cases alternative drugs can be prescribed with less severe side-effects, but until the drugs have been tried no one knows just how the patient will respond.

For example, some women experience headaches, nausea or bleeding problems with certain types of Pill. Changing brands can get rid of the problem. The same goes for anti-arthritic and blood-pressure-lowering drugs but you probably need to give them a proper try before assuming the side-effects are too unpleasant to put up with.

If the doctor warned us about every possible side-effect of a drug we were prescribed we would never even take the prescription to the chemist to get it made up! The textbooks contain reports of extremely rare side-effects such as blood disorders or kidney failure with even the most commonly used drugs. But these effects are incredibly rare and may be only indirectly related to using the drug, or the patient may have had some unusual illness which made him or her prone to that particular side-effect.

In some cases it is important that patients should be warned not to take other drugs while on a particular medicine. Just as you should not eat cheese with antidepressants or take some antibiotics with milk, some medicines should not be taken together. Hundreds of these so-called drug interactions have been documented. Many are of little more than academic interest. But others are important. Some drugs increase, and some decrease, the potency of other medicines and this may mean that doses have to be adapted accordingly. Alternatively, some drugs may make side-effects of other drugs worse when they are taken together.

If you are worried about side-effects or interactions between drugs, ask the doctor how commonly they occur and whether there is anything you can do to avoid them. And, as in the case of the information about your illness, the dose of your medicine and how long you should take it, ask the doctor to write down the side-effects for you if you think you will get confused about them. You probably will not want to write down what the doctor tells you in the surgery – although there is no reason why you should not. But as soon as you get outside you can jot down what has been said to you before you have a chance to forget. Or if you are with someone tell them what the doctor has said and ask them to help you remember.

There is a move towards drugs being dispensed with information leaflets explaining how to take them. Unfortunately progress has been slow and it could be some years before leaflets are widely available.

Information Leaflets

In Britain the only drug which is routinely accompanied by an information leaflet for patients is the contraceptive pill. In the United States and Canada dozens of drugs have leaflets, each approved by the health authorities.

Other drug manufacturers in Britain do voluntarily provide

information leaflets with their drugs, but if they decide to do so, they have, by law, to supply details of the dangers of their drug more suited to a medical than a lay readership. Each side-effect, however rare, must be itemized – to startling effect for the untrained eye.

Faced with a double sheet of closely typed information, few patients actually read the leaflets provided. Yet if they were produced in more readable form such leaflets could not only enable patients to take their medicine more effectively but could also allay many of the worries experienced by patients – particularly when they are taking a drug for the first time.

The question of how much to tell patients both verbally and in written form is hotly debated. And the case of Amy Siddaway, the woman who sued her surgeon for not telling her that an operation on her neck might leave her partially paralysed, highlighted the difficulties faced by doctors and patients over their choices of treatment. Mrs Siddaway lost her case because it was established that she was told what current medical thinking accepts was sufficient for her case. In other words, other surgeons, faced with a similar type of case, would also have failed to warn of the particular risk Mrs Siddaway was taking.

What befell Mrs Siddaway was a rare condition roughly akin to some of the equally rare but potentially very serious blood disorders which are known to occur with some drugs. Should patients be told about these or can they be passed off simply as exceptionally rare? Various systems have been proposed for presenting information to patients and some of these have already been incorporated in leaflets produced abroad.

Doctors and sociologists at Southampton University are currently assessing the pros and cons of a series of leaflets they have designed for patients taking common drugs such as penicillins, anti-arthritic and antihypertensive agents. Each leaflet makes five basic points:

– make sure that there is no reason why you should not be taking the drug,
– check the label on the medicine for instructions about how to take it,
– take the course as prescribed,

– keep your medicine out of reach of children,
– dispose of any drugs you do not use.

So how important are these points?

Most patients can take most drugs. But there are always a few patients who are either allergic to the drugs or have reacted badly to them in the past. Doctors should be aware of this. But patients do not always see their own doctor and the allergy to a drug may be hidden deep in the notes. If you know you are allergic to penicillin or are prone to stomach problems with aspirin it is important to mention this so that the doctor can prescribe something which will suit you.

Of course, by the time you get an information leaflet which tells you to be wary of taking drugs to which you might be allergic you have probably already got the drugs. But it is a fail-safe device, so that if you are worried you can go back to your doctor or ring and check that it is safe to take them.

The Southampton leaflets also include information about common side-effects. One way round the problem of what to tell patients might be to grade side-effects according to whether you should grin and bear it or go straight to your doctor. But would this be alarmist, and could patients panic if their side-effect fell in the second category? It is hard to tell, and inevitably there are people who will worry more than others. Another option would be to grade side-effects according to frequency. So that if you found nausea was one of the most common side-effects you would know not to worry, but if you experienced something rare you could tell your doctor. The problem with this approach is that not everything which is common is safe nor is every rare side-effect dangerous. So it may be better to take the approach which advises patients to go to their doctor if they experience one of a series of side-effects known to be more dangerous.

Drug Labels

The label on your medicine should contain the following information:

– the name of the drug,
– the dose of the drug and how often to take it,

– any important warnings, for example, 'not to be taken in pregnancy' if it is a drug which will harm an unborn baby.

Unfortunately this information is not required by law and is frequently missing, though pharmacists do now provide more information than previously.

Time and again, studies have shown that people who do not understand the directions for their medicines fail to take them properly. Between a quarter and a half of all patients either do not take their medicine at all or take it incorrectly. And the worst offenders are those on longer-term treatment – just the ones who need it most. Not only do people take their medicines incorrectly, but they store them away for years. A study of 192 homes carried out a few years ago showed that the average medicine cabinet contains three bottles or packets of prescribed medicines. Some 28 per cent of these medicines were never taken and only half were in current use.

Storing Medicines

Storage and disposal of medicines is important. Drugs, like food, go off and the length of time they remain active varies enormously. Creams in tubs and eye drops are likely to decay most quickly. Ointments in tubes keep for a little longer. Antibiotics should never be kept after a course of treatment and aspirin and paracetamol should be thrown away as soon as they smell vinegary. Pre-packed drugs often carry a 'use by' date, which should be strictly adhered to. Other medicines may not carry an expiry date, but the basic message is: if you no longer need it, throw it away.

Storage of medicines is also important. You would not keep bread or cheese in a steamy bathroom so why subject your medicines to such conditions? All medicines should be kept at or just below average room temperature, away from extremes of heat, sunlight or dampness. That is not to say that medicines will decompose at the first dribble of condensation down the wall. They are designed to withstand reasonable variations in temperature. But if mistreated over long periods they are likely to become less effective.

It is one thing to use up a bottle of cough mixture on someone in the same family with a similar type of cough to the one for which the medicine was bought. It is quite another to use up prescribed medicines because someone in the family appears to have a similar type of stomach upset or respiratory infection. It may be dangerous to do so. For example, someone who is regularly given antibiotics he does not need may build up a resistance to them which may make them ineffective when he does get an infection.

Some tablets suit one patient and not another. The contraceptive pill is perfectly safe for most women but not for someone with high blood pressure. A beta-blocker for high blood pressure is perfectly safe for most people with palpitations, but not for an asthmatic. And so it goes on.

Every year hospitals deal with around 200,000 admissions of people who have been poisoned by drugs or other household products. The majority are children who have somehow managed to get hold of adult medicines. Most recently there has been an increase in the number of children who have taken their mothers' contraceptive pills. This is because medicines are frequently left around, not least as a reminder for patients to take them. Children, having seen their parents take the medicine, follow suit. All medicine should be kept out of reach of children. Put a reminder on your jotting-pad or leave an empty bottle out as a reminder, but not the real thing.

Where Should Information Be Available?

In Britain we have been slow to develop the idea of providing people with leaflets about their drugs. The government and other grant-giving bodies have made small amounts of money available to test a leaflet system but progress has been slow. Follow-up interviews with people in the Southampton area given leaflets about their drugs have shown that people do remember more about their drugs if verbal information is backed up by written leaflets, and this both enables them to take their medicine more effectively and reduces their worries about their drugs.

As yet, the handing out of information leaflets has been the domain of the doctor but many believe that the leaflets should be available at the point where the patient picks up his medicine – at the chemist's shop. The pharmacist could hand over the drugs with a few words of advice on taking them and reinforce his advice with a leaflet.

Some people may not feel as confident about information given by their pharmacist as by their doctor and it is vital that both professionals give out the same information; otherwise the patient would be truly baffled. Yet the highly trained pharmacist is well informed about the doses of drugs, what side-effects to look out for and the drugs which should not be taken at the same time.

Ironically, this debate – where the information leaflets should be available – may become academic with the spread of increasing numbers of drugs being dispensed in the original packaging in which they left the factory. Instead of pharmacists transferring medicines from large cartons to small individual bottles they will soon dispense virtually all medicines in unopened packages of twenty, fifty or one hundred tablets, as required. It then becomes much easier for patients to be given leaflets with their medicines.

When this does become the norm, it will be important that doctors do not neglect their role in the dispersal of information. Simply to tell patients that instructions on their use will be in the packaging of drugs would be counter-productive. For though most people read the instructions on how to use a new radio or television, they expect some form of demonstration first in the shop. And so it is with medicines. It is the job of both doctor and pharmacist to give preliminary information about drugs, and information leaflets should remain a back-up.

It is hoped that when leaflets are routinely included in drug packaging they will contain the information patients need. If they consist of a closely typed leaflet of information which the drug company is using to protect itself against claims of negligence, then they will do little to help the patient to take his medicine correctly.

CHAPTER 3

Are Drugs Safe?

Got a pain? Take a pill. Sore throat? Suck a pastille. Upset stomach? Drink this. It is not surprising that we expect so much from our drugs. Newspapers, books and television tell us about the latest breakthrough, the newest drugs. Why suffer in silence when drugs can soothe your head, your stomach, your aching heart? But nothing comes free. There is a price to pay for these supposed cure-alls. Each time we take a drug we expect two things – that it will work and that it is safe. But are we right to make such assumptions?

Every day we take risks, consciously or unconsciously, at work, in our homes, walking down the street. Few of us could put a figure on those risks but we know, in general terms, that we are more likely to be killed in a road accident than to be struck by lightning, more likely to have a fatal accident if we go mountaineering than if we sit in front of the television, and at greater risk if we work in the construction industry than if we stay in an office.

We know the ground rules; we take risks and we do not live in fear of the consequences. But when it comes to drugs we rarely know what the risks are, let alone whether they are worth taking. Only thirteen of the 2000-odd recorded deaths caused by everyday medicines in 1983 in the United Kingdom occurred when normal doses were taken. Around 400 of these deaths resulted from accidental overdoses and all the rest were suicides. By comparison an estimated 100,000 people die from smoking-related deaths each year, 8000 from alcohol abuse and 4000 in motor accidents.

But it is always the unknown risks which worry us most and, while drugs may not kill very often, they can make us feel very ill; an estimated one in twenty admissions to hospital are related to problems with drugs – not the addictive drugs with a capital

'D' but the everyday drugs prescribed by doctors or bought from chemists.

All drugs have unwanted as well as beneficial effects and, in general, the more serious the illness being treated the more severe the side-effects of the drugs. Some side-effects are worth putting up with because of the overall benefit brought by the drug; others are not. It is a question of weighing the benefits against the risks of the drug and this balance will shift according to the severity of the disease.

Many people who take drugs to control their blood pressure put up with feeling tired or sick when they take their medicine. That is because if their blood pressure goes very high they risk having a heart attack. Some arthritic patients suffer from indigestion when they take drugs to soothe their swollen joints but they consider it a small price to pay for remaining active, mobile and free of pain. But even these fairly minor problems would be too high a price for someone who just wanted to be rid of a headache. If they were very severe, they would even become unacceptable to the patients with high blood pressure and arthritis. Ultimately, people with the most serious diseases, such as cancer, put up with very unpleasant side-effects from their drugs because they would die without them.

How long you have to take a drug will also influence whether it is worth putting up with the side-effects. Many people are prepared to feel sick or tired for a day or two but would have second thoughts about those side-effects if they had to take the medicine for months or years. Striking a balance becomes even more difficult for someone who is perfectly healthy but needs a drug for some other reason. Women taking the contraceptive pill fall into this category.

Another dilemma faces someone trying to decide whether to take drugs to prevent rather than cure an illness. Most of us have had a typhoid injection before going on holiday and the spread of the disease into package-holiday areas such as the Mediterranean has meant that more people than ever are being advised to have the injection. Everyone responds differently to such injections. Some get mild cold symptoms, others may feel unwell for two or three days. But compared to the disease, these side-effects are very minor and most people are prepared to put up with them.

In these cases, we are making the decisions for ourselves. But what happens when we are making them for someone else? Most children are vaccinated routinely against a variety of infections – tuberculosis, polio, diphtheria, German measles. But nowhere has there been more debate than over the routine immunization of children against whooping cough. Far less controversy hangs over whether pregnant women should take medicines. In the wake of the thalidomide tragedy women are now advised to take drugs only if really necessary during pregnancy, especially during the first few months when organ formation occurs.

All decisions about taking drugs should be taken with a knowledge of the issues involved. We are not doctors, we do not have a detailed knowledge of drugs, but we can understand the factors which influence the balance between risk and benefit. And we must take part in deciding what is acceptable to us – the risks which are worth taking, and those which are not.

Sean is 15 and has had asthma since he was a baby. Today, he takes one drug four times a day to prevent asthma attacks and a second drug to relieve symptoms if he starts getting wheezy. He plays football with his friends, rides his bike and has won medals for fishing.

'My asthma doesn't stop me from doing what I want to do. I carry my inhaler around with me and if I feel an attack coming on I use it. One or two puffs and I'm usually better.'

Without his asthma drugs there is no doubt that Sean could not lead the active boy's life he does. He wouldn't be able to play games at school and the first puff of wind would send him indoors.

'I don't know what would happen without the drugs. I suppose I would just go on and on wheezing.'

Lynn's little boy, Benjamin, has been prescribed drugs for his eczema since he was a baby. But she has never been told what they are or what is in them.

'It's very difficult as a parent to question the doctor. You want your child to get better as quickly as possible and you are not prepared to take the risks with his health which you might take with your own. You feel that you cannot question whether he really needs them or if they have side-effects.'

Lynn knew the sorts of questions she should ask about the drugs her son was taking, but as soon as she got into the doctor's surgery she found it very difficult to ask them. She therefore played no part in deciding whether the benefits of the medicine outweighed the risks which might go with them.

Making Decisions

Drugs for high blood pressure

Millions of people all over the world take drugs to control their blood pressure. They take them two or three times a day, every day of the year and they may find themselves on therapy for the rest of their lives. Depending on the levels of their raised blood pressure they risk fatigue, palpitations and even heart attack or stroke if they fail to take their medicine.

Two types of drug are commonly taken for blood pressure. Beta-blockers relax the heart and hence reduce the pressure of blood flowing through the blood vessels. Diuretics act on the kidney to increase the amount of water extracted from the blood and passed in the urine, thus decreasing blood volume and hence pressure.

Both drugs have unwanted effects. Beta-blockers can cause tiredness, nausea, insomnia, a slowing of the heart beat, and poor circulation to the limbs. Diuretics inevitably cause a significant increase in the amount of urine passed since this is how they work to reduce blood pressure. More significantly they cause a reduction in the body's potassium supplies which can have a serious effect on the electrical activity of the heart.

Numerous studies have been carried out to try and pinpoint the precise level of blood pressure above which there is an increased risk of heart attack. But as yet there is no answer. When patients' blood pressure is so high that they are aware of symptoms there is little choice. They must risk the side-effects of drugs in order to lower pressure and reduce their risk of serious illness. But, where their blood pressure is only slightly raised, is the risk of side-effects worth taking? If lowering the blood pressure is not going to affect their chances of a heart attack should people have to put up with sleepless nights, feeling sick or loss of libido. (Interestingly, it has only been through the studies of blood pressure that it was discovered that one commonly used beta-blocker is an effective contraceptive!) There seems little point in treating one relatively mild condition only to give patients side-effects which themselves require drug treatment. Preventive measures such as losing weight, stopping smoking and reducing salt intake may be more appropriate.

Jim was to have gone on holiday the day after he had his heart attack. It started when he got home from work, tired and breathless. The pain in his chest got worse and the doctor sent him straight to hospital. When the immediate danger was over Jim's doctor prescribed three different drugs to keep his heart and blood pressure steady.

At first all went well. But after a few months Jim found himself getting more and more tired. The short walk to the station to get to work was almost too much for him and even the lightest jobs at home were out of the question. Jim's wife took over mowing the lawn.

Initially the doctor thought that Jim might be heading for another heart attack. But tests at the hospital showed that all was well, and since tiredness can be a side-effect of the beta-blocker which was amongst Jim's medication, the doctor advised him to stop taking it. The effect was immediate.

'I won't say I turned into a spring chicken but the tiredness got less and I now feel a hundred per cent better. I can get to the station without having to stop and I can do the garden and jobs around the house without any problem,' said Jim.

Jim's doctor was well aware that stopping the beta-blocker might deprive Jim of some long-term protection against a second heart attack. But as taking the drug left Jim constantly tired and depressed, the doctor felt that in this case the benefits of the medicine simply did not outweigh the side-effects.

Kenneth went to his GP with a routine ear infection. But his doctor decided to do a quick check on his blood pressure as well. To everyone's surprise his blood pressure was slightly high, and it was still at the same level when it was measured again the following week.

The doctor recommended that Kenneth should start a course of treatment with a beta-blocker to reduce his blood pressure.

'I must say I wasn't very keen on the idea, particularly when the doctor said I would probably have to take them for the rest of my life and I didn't feel ill in any way. But I trust my doctor and so I decided to go ahead with them. I've had no problems with the drugs and I feel fine,' said Kenneth.

There is some evidence that lowering blood pressure with beta-blockers can reduce the risk of later heart problems. Kenneth had no symptoms when the medicine was prescribed, but his doctor was looking to the future.

Diabetes

This is another disease which requires chronic treatment but the benefits of treatment more obviously outweigh the risk. At its most severe, too much sugar in the blood will send the patient into coma and probable death. Without properly controlled levels of blood sugar, patients risk blindness, severe nervous and kidney diseases and gangrene of the hands and feet caused by poor circulation to the extremities.

Placed alongside the discomfort of insulin injections, the inconvenience of diets and the nausea, indigestion and other gastric problems which can accompany some anti-diabetic drugs, the choice is obvious.

Cancer

No patients have to put up with more unpleasant side-effects than those undergoing treatment for cancer. Sadly, cytotoxic drugs used to kill tumours are not sufficiently specific to avoid killing normal cells and many of the side-effects of these drugs can be attributed to their effects on normal, healthy cells. During and immediately after cancer chemotherapy most patients are very sick; they feel exhausted and ill. They lose their appetite and within a few days they frequently develop severe mouth ulcers that make it hard to eat even if they have the appetite. Most of these drugs suppress the immune cells in the blood, leaving patients open to infections and other serious illnesses. Many anti-cancer drugs can also cause the patient's hair to fall out because the drugs kill the hair cells. With a limited number of drugs, wrapping the head in ice packs during treatment can prevent hair loss because it prevents the drug getting at the roots of the hair. But without this treatment most patients lose some or all of their hair.

The total effect is very debilitating and demoralizing but, where the alternative is almost certain death, few cancer patients balk at the unenviable choice between treatment and no treatment. In no other instance is the option so poor that patients are prepared to put up with this sort of level of side-effects. In this case even these enormous risks may be outweighed by the possible benefits.

Again, the balance depends on the probable outcome. Some forms of cancer such as Hodgkin's disease, testicular and ovarian cancers, some leukaemias and some breast and lung tumours do respond well to anti-cancer drugs: in fact, a cure is a reasonable prospect and the side-effects of the drugs worth bearing. But in other forms of cancer, drugs can do little to improve the outcome and patients may be made miserable in their last months by the side-effects of their drugs. In all these cases, patients should be offered the facts and allowed to decide for themselves, if they wish.

Vicky's ovarian cancer was diagnosed when she was in her thirties. A doctor herself, specializing in hormone research, she suddenly realized how little she knew about cancer. Initially, she had surgery to remove the tumour, followed by a course of intensive drug treatment to stamp out any remaining cancer cells.

'The treatment was very unpleasant. I was sick, my hair fell out and I felt very ill. But I was determined to do everything to improve my chances of surviving,' Vicky said.

Apparently free from cancer, Vicky went back to work, only to discover soon afterwards that it had recurred. Further surgery and drug therapy followed, as well as some of the very latest cancer treatment. Another year followed and yet more treatment was needed.

Four years after her cancer was diagnosed, Vicky had had

virtually every type of treatment available – each with its own horrible side-effects. But Vicky has no regrets.

'I kept setting myself targets – first to live six months, then a year, and so on. I cannot look very far ahead but I'm trying to pack as much into my life now as possible. I would not be here without the treatments I have had, so the side-effects must have been worth it.'

Rosamond's lung cancer was diagnosed just over a year after her husband had died from cancer of the intestine. Having seen the effects of cancer she was only too aware of the dangers. On the advice of her doctors she agreed to a course of chemotherapy to treat her tumour and try to prevent it spreading.

She went into hospital for two days each month for treatment, which made her sick so that she could not eat. After each treatment she developed painful mouth ulcers, and she felt tired and depressed. After a couple of months her hair started to fall out; eventually she lost it all and wore a wig.

The drugs did halt the progress of the tumour and Rosamond spent a Christmas with her family which her children had thought she would not see. But by this time Rosamond had found the side-effects of her treatment too much to bear and it was stopped.

Rosamond died four months later, two years to the day after her husband. Almost certainly, the drug she was given had prolonged her life by six months. But her children remained unsure of whether the extra months had been worth the side-effects caused by the treatment. Their mother had a strong will to survive, but never really knew how ill she was or that the drugs were only postponing the inevitable outcome.

Contraception

The first hormone contraceptive pills came on to the market in the late 1950s and early 1960s and early side-effects from the high doses of hormones quickly led to a drop in dose. But it was not until the early 1970s that the first research began to link the Pill with an increased risk of thrombosis. It was decided that oestrogen was the culprit and the dose reduced once more. A few years later it was the turn of the progestogen component of the Pill and this time it seemed to be arterial diseases which were more common in Pill users.

Meanwhile it was shown that it was only older women and in particular those who smoked who seemed to be at increased risk of circulatory problems. Provided women had their blood pressure measured regularly, doctors could watch for those showing such problems.

Things went quiet for a few years. The hormone content of the Pill was at its lowest level. It was still the most effective form of contraception available and it seemed that if you were not in one of the high-risk groups – that is, you were not over thirty-five, did not smoke and you were not overweight – you would be all right. If women needed any more reason to go back to the Pill they were given it by a worrying increase in pelvic infection and infertility in women using the only other really effective method of contraception – the intrauterine device (IUD).

Then came a new scare, this time far more frightening than arterial disease – cancer. Two papers published in the autumn of 1983 linked the Pill with both breast and cervical cancer. The methods used in the breast-cancer study were later questioned but the link with cervical cancer remains; indeed, last year a further paper implicated the Pill. True, the Pill appears actually to protect against ovarian cancer and tumours of the body of the womb – two particularly lethal forms of the disease – but the link with cervical cancer stuck. An estimated half a million women stopped taking the Pill after the first Pill scare, and the abortion rate rose in the nine months following the 1983 cancer scare, though no one can be sure that this was because women threw away their Pills.

Faced with the knowledge of the last two decades, women wanting effective contraception have to make a far more difficult choice today than their mothers thirty years ago, who were among the first to take the Pill and who were, together with their doctors, totally ignorant of the possible dangers of the drug. The Pill is almost 100 per cent effective. This compares with around 97 per cent effectiveness for the sheath or cap when used with spermicide – and that is for the most careful users; figures are far lower when these methods are not used properly.

The risks of death or serious illness from childbirth or abortion are very small. But the social upheaval of an unwanted child also has to be considered in the overall risks-versus-benefits equation of using the Pill.

Current advice would be this. If you do not smoke, you are not overweight, there is no heart disease in your family and you have your blood pressure checked regularly there is no reason why you should not go on taking the Pill. Some authorities even argue that these lowest-risk women can continue taking it until they are menopausal. If you do smoke, are overweight, or have one or more of the other 'risk' factors you would be advised to stop smoking and lose weight or consider alternative methods of contraception after the age of thirty to thirty-five. If you have already had children the IUD is one alternative; if you have completed your family then vasectomy or sterilization is another.

It is still not possible to make definite recommendations to take account of the cancer risks, not least because the studies carried out to date have included women on Pills containing higher levels of hormones than used in today's Pills. But some preventive measures can be taken. Regular smears, every three to five years, can pick up the first pre-cancerous stages of cervical cancer and regular breast examination can help find lumps before they have a chance to spread.

By taking all these factors and checks into consideration the woman on the Pill can shift the weight of her own risk–benefit equation strongly in her favour and minimize the risks to her health. Before making her decision to start or stay on the Pill she should know the facts as they relate to her health in order to make her decision from a point of understanding rather than ignorance.

Jill is in her early thirties; she does not smoke but she would like to lose a few pounds in weight. She has been taking the contraceptive pill on and off for over ten years. She is single, has a good job, owns her own house and has a steady boyfriend. Eventually she might want children, but at present they don't fit in with her career plans.

'I decided to stay on the Pill in spite of all the scare stories because it suits me. I feel fine, it is convenient and there is no risk of me getting pregnant. I am aware that the risks of thrombosis do increase as a woman gets older. But I don't smoke and my blood pressure is always normal. So why should I give up?'

Jill's doctor agrees that since she is at relatively small risk of thrombosis she should stay on the Pill and not worry about changing to another method of contraception. If she smoked, was very overweight or had a history of circulatory problems, her doctor would almost certainly advise differently.

Ann is also in her early thirties; she does not smoke and is tall and slim – not an obvious target for circulatory problems. But after six years of taking the contraceptive pill, Ann recently came off it because her blood pressure had gone up.

'My doctor suggested that I consider some alternative method of contraception because of the blood pressure problem. I tried changing brands of Pill but my blood pressure would not come down.'

Married with two children, Ann is now considering sterilization, since she has not got on well with the other methods of contraception she has tried and she does not want any more children.

'I would have preferred to stay on the Pill and not have the sterilization, and I still haven't decided finally what to do. But my blood pressure certainly stopped me from continuing with the Pill.'

Immunization

If making a decision which affects your own health seems difficult, a decision affecting someone dear to you can be much more difficult. One such decision affects most parents trying to decide whether to have their child vaccinated against whooping cough.

The number of children who get whooping cough each year varies enormously, from under 20,000 in a good year, to over 60,000 during an epidemic. Most children first feel feverish, and then get the cough after which the disease is named. During the 1977–9 epidemic, when 102,000 children caught the infection, 5000 were admitted to hospital and twenty-seven died. A further seventeen suffered permanent brain damage.

Government policy is to encourage parents to have their children immunized against whooping cough by the time they are three years old, and at present about 55 per cent of parents take this advice. This compares with around 80 per cent before the

1970s scare over immunization, after which immunization levels fell to 31 per cent, quickly followed by an epidemic of the infection. Official estimates put the risk of brain damage from whooping-cough vaccine at about one in 100,000 children, equivalent to about four children a year. But pressure groups campaigning on behalf of parents of vaccine-damaged children believe that the risks from whooping-cough vaccines are far greater.

The government has set up a fund for children where there is strong evidence that they have been permanently damaged by vaccination of any sort. When cases are proved, children get a payment of £10,000 but only about one in four claims have been granted awards of money. In many other cases it was felt that damage was not related to the vaccine or that the disability was not sufficiently severe to merit a payment. The Association of Parents of Vaccine Damaged Children is trying to get better settlements for children they believe have been damaged, by taking their cases through the courts, as they do not feel that a one-off payment of £10,000 is sufficient to provide lifelong care for those who have been disabled.

Most vaccines cause some minor side-effects; this is to be expected, as the patient is being introduced to the organism which is capable of causing the disease. In the vaccine, the organism may have been killed or may be present in such small quantities that it causes only minor symptoms. But we have all experienced symptoms of fever and malaise after a typhoid injection or an influenza vaccination. Research is under way to provide a safer whooping-cough vaccine that will be less likely to cause serious side-effects. But, until then, parents must assess the risk of their child being damaged by the vaccine against the chances of serious illness if he contracts the infection.

A decision on whooping-cough vaccine is possibly the most difficult drug decision to make. The disease is not a 'life or death' one like cancer, it is not a highly dangerous condition like uncontrolled diabetes or high blood pressure; it is not even possible to isolate 'high-risk groups', as in the case of women trying to decide whether to take the contraceptive pill, though there are some children for whom it is definitely not recommended. Yet it is a decision facing thousands of parents each year. A safer vaccine is the only real answer to the dilemma.

James was just a few months old when his parents made the difficult decision to have him vaccinated against whooping cough. James's mother, Ruth, had been a primary school teacher and had seen the effects of whooping cough on children in her class.

'One child in particular was very bad. He was off school for eight weeks and the following term he still seemed to be suffering the after-effects – catching one thing after another. We didn't want James to have to go through that,' said Ruth. But in the back of her mind was the risk of brain damage from the whooping-cough vaccine.

'I had read about the dangers of the vaccine and I knew I would never forgive myself if he was damaged. We were aware that we were making a decision on his behalf and that before the vaccine he was a normal healthy baby. I could not take my eyes off him in the first few hours after he had the whooping-cough vaccine.'

James suffered no ill effects from the vaccine.

Simon's parents also thought long and hard before agreeing to have him vaccinated against whooping cough. Like Ruth and her husband, they had been warned that an epidemic had been predicted for the start of 1986. They decided to give him the vaccine. A few weeks after his first injection Simon started coughing badly.

'It was only when the doctor finally heard him coughing in the surgery that he said that Simon had in fact got whooping cough. We were told that it could not have resulted from the vaccine itself but that the infection would probably have been worse if he had not been vaccinated. It was quite bad enough as it was, so we were very glad that we had gone ahead,' said Simon's mother.

Drugs in pregnancy

Medical opinion is far less divided over whether women should take drugs in pregnancy than it is over whooping-cough vaccination. 'If you can possibly avoid it do not take any drug when you are pregnant, especially in the first three months', is the basic message currently given to pregnant women. Following the thalidomide tragedy of the 1960s, doctors have become increasingly aware of the danger of drugs, taken by pregnant women, passing across the placenta and either causing deformities or slowing the rate of growth of the foetus. Cigarettes and alcohol also count as drugs in this context and large amounts of caffeine are best avoided.

Pregnant women should think twice about taking drugs even before they know they are pregnant. The first six to eight weeks of a pregnancy – frequently a time when women do not even know that a baby is on the way – are amongst the most crucial of the pregnancy. So women who are no longer using contraceptives and are trying to have a baby should consider themselves 'pregnant' as far as drugs, alcohol and smoking are concerned.

Of course, there are exceptions. Diabetics, epileptics and women with high blood pressure are three groups for whom drug-taking in pregnancy is probably inevitable. The complications of these chronic diseases would be much more dangerous to an unborn baby than the possible side-effects of the drugs used to control symptoms. Any woman planning to have a baby who takes medicine for a chronic illness, be it migraine or asthma, high blood pressure or eczema should discuss fully her drugs, and their side-effects, with her doctor before attempting to become pregnant.

Medicines for the elderly

If the unborn child is at greatest risk of drug injury, then those at the other end of the age spectrum cannot be far behind. The elderly account for over a third of medicines dispensed by the NHS and, at thirteen prescriptions a year, they consume double the national average number of prescriptions. Not only are they at greater risk of drug injury because of the sheer quantities of medicines they take, but their slower metabolism of drugs also makes them vulnerable.

The liver and kidneys of elderly people are less efficient at breaking down and getting rid of drugs than younger people's. So medicines can build up in their bodies, sometimes with devastating effect. Many of those who are thought to have died from liver and kidney diseases after taking the anti-arthritic drug, Opren, are thought to have accumulated the drug in their bodies and they probably needed far lower doses than were prescribed.

Drugs behave differently in the elderly from the moment they go into the patient's mouth. The elderly gut moves more slowly than a younger one, leaving more time for drugs to be absorbed across the intestine. Greater absorption means that more drug gets into the bloodstream. The liver is responsible for breaking down, metabolizing and excreting some drugs. If it is not fully functional, drugs tend to accumulate and this is particularly common with certain tranquillizers and sleeping pills. The kidney is generally the final excretor of drugs and since people in their eighties have only about 60 per cent of the kidney filtration capacity of a younger person, drugs are excreted more slowly. Many older people take several different types of drug and not only do these compete for the limited liver and kidney function available, they can also interact with each other.

On top of the physical problems which the elderly have in dealing with their drugs, they also have difficulty in remembering to take them regularly and correctly. It is inevitable that the more drugs people take, the harder it becomes to remember them all. In addition, the elderly generally draw the short straw when it comes to getting information about their drugs in the first place. If they are housebound, they may get the information second- or third-hand from whoever collects their drugs for them and many are locked into the repeat-prescription system, which may mean that they do not see their doctor often enough to ask questions about dosage or the side-effects they may be experiencing.

Doctors are increasingly being advised to reduce the number of drugs they prescribe to elderly people. They are also being asked to lower the dose. Thus the maximum dose of the tranquillizer diazepam that is recommended for the elderly is half that recommended for a healthy adult. Experts recommend that, in general, the initial dose of a drug when prescribed for an elderly person should be half that normally given to an adult. If the patient does not respond, the dose can be slowly stepped up. But starting on a low dose may reduce the number of drug problems experienced by the elderly.

Mysterious or apparently unrelated side-effects reported by an elderly patient should always be taken seriously. Because some elderly patients appear confused, it does not mean they cannot recognize something odd which is happening to them and may be related to their drugs.

A number of methods have been designed to help elderly patients remember to take their medicines. One of the best systems is a container for the drugs with slots marked off, containing tablets to be taken at specific times. Both the patient, and the health visitor, or relative, can see at a glance whether the medicines are up to date. Large charts with the time of day to take different-coloured tablets can also help, especially if there is a space for the patient to tick off when the medicine has been taken. Another alternative is a musical pill-box which 'plays' at set times of day – but this is only useful if the patient is taking one medicine and has good hearing.

It is inevitable that elderly people will need more medicines than younger people but a little extra care from the doctor in prescribing, and from friends and relatives in ensuring that the patient takes the medicines correctly, can reduce the risk of drug accidents.

Following the Opren tragedy, the government has introduced new rules which insist that any new medicine which is likely to be taken by older people should be tested on people of that age group before it is marketed. In this way it is hoped that the correct dose, and any particular side-effects likely to be experienced by the elderly, will be recognized before rather than after the drug is licensed.

CHAPTER 4

Testing New Drugs

In the wake of the thalidomide disaster a system for testing all new drugs was set up to ensure their safety and effectiveness. Until the 1968 Medicines Act, there was no legal requirement for drug companies to test their products. The series of animal and human tests which have since evolved are not foolproof. Drugs do still slip through the net. Witness Opren, Flosint, Zelmid, Zomax – all drugs which had to be withdrawn within a few years of being licensed. No drug can be guaranteed free from side-effects though many of the unwanted effects of older drugs would not be tolerated in new products. Just how are these drugs tested and do we have any guarantees that another thalidomide could not come on the market?

Designing a new drug is like talent-spotting. You can find a product which looks good and performs well but only a tiny minority of them have that extra something which gives them star quality. Every new drug which comes on to the market will have taken up to ten years of research and development in laboratories and hospitals. As many as 10,000 chemicals will have been scrutinized and discarded in the search for that elusive 'new' drug. Very few even make it off the starting-blocks. An enormous amount of information on potential new drugs is stored on computers. A quick scan of the data-banks will show that the vast majority of chemicals available are not worth considering. They may be difficult to make or too expensive; they may be unstable, ineffective or likely to have serious side-effects. In addition to drawing on the vast stores of information gleaned from previous drug research, scientists can assess some potential new drugs without reaching for a test tube. They can use computers to put pictures of chemicals on screen and see how well they would bind to receptor sites on the tissues if they were real drugs.

Once the initial choice of thousands of chemicals has been

narrowed to only a few hundred, a chemist can set about making some of them ready for the first laboratory tests. Again, all kinds of unforeseen problems can arise which will make any further tests a waste of time. Finally, armed with perhaps thirty chemicals, the pharmacologist and biochemist can begin the laboratory tests which provide the first information about how a drug works. The most promising of this batch of drugs begin tests on animals. Specially bred rats and mice are most commonly used for these experiments, which centre initially on assessing the toxicity of each new drug.

At present this involves one of the most controversial tests used for animal studies. It is called the LD 50 test. Quite simply, a batch of animals are given increasing doses of the new drug until half of them are dead. The dose which causes this 50 per cent mortality is then recorded and can be compared with that required for other similar drugs. Both health officials and scientists in Britain are unhappy about such a test which is expensive in animals and gives only the broadest information about a drug's dangers. Proposals to do away with the LD 50 test are being considered by EEC legislators but, in spite of general agreement that the test is unnecessary, delays have meant that companies still perform the test.

Even if the LD 50 test is removed, other toxicity tests will remain, until checks are developed which can be carried out without animals. Already, research is under way to develop more accurate tests which do not require live animals. Apart from anything else, animals respond to drugs differently from humans and so more accurate tests are needed.

Scientists are developing methods which use isolated cells (rather than whole animals) to test drugs. A major project set up by FRAME (Fund for the Replacement of Animals in Medical Experiments) is currently assessing whether a battery of tests using bacterial, animal and human cells grown in the laboratory can give as accurate information on drug safety as conventional animal experiments. It is unlikely that any one such test will replace animal studies altogether, but a battery of these tests using different types of cell could give an accurate guide to drug safety.

Similar tests are already being used routinely to test the

mutagenicity of a drug, that is, its capacity to alter the genetic material in the cell. Such changes could have long-term consequences to the health of both the individual who takes the drug and his or her children.

But with the exception of these mutation tests, much of the early experimentation with drugs is performed on animals. In addition to the immediate toxicity of the drug, scientists must check its potential to cause cancer or to affect the subsequent fertility of the test animals. Also they must ascertain the effects of the drug on pregnant animals to ensure that it cannot damage the unborn baby.

Some of these tests are done alongside each other; others, the long-term and generally more expensive tests, are done after the first experiments with the new drug on humans. It is only in the last few years that drug companies have been allowed to begin their human tests before completing all the animal experiments. It was considered unfair that they should expend vast amounts of time and money performing lengthy cancer and other tests before the most important question of all had been answered. Would the drug work in humans? All the safety testing in the world would be of no use if the drug did not actually work on the subjects for whom it was intended. So now the first human studies are done before the animal tests are completed.

It may seem curious but the first human tests of a new drug are done on perfectly healthy human volunteers. Frequently these tests are carried out on people who actually work for the drug company developing the new drug. Where there is goodwill between employers and staff there is likely to be a ready supply of volunteers. In the event of an accident or emergency, expert advice is on hand. Regular monitoring of blood and other samples from the volunteers is also simplified if they are working at the same site as that where the experiments are carried out.

Drug companies are encouraged to submit plans for these volunteer studies to ethical committees which are set up nationwide to check that trials are justifiable on both scientific and ethical grounds. These committees are composed of scientists and professional laymen, such as lawyers and accountants. However, two recent deaths of healthy volunteers in drug trials have highlighted anomalies in the system. In 1983 a Dublin man dropped dead shortly after he was given a new heart drug and in the same year a Welsh medical student died as a result of an immune disorder after taking a new tranquillizer.

The Royal College of Physicians (RCP) has conducted an inquiry into the rights and protection of volunteers for human studies on behalf of the Medicines Commission attached to the Department of Health and Social Security (DHSS). All subjects must at present give their informed consent to participate in a study. But just how much are volunteers told about the drug which they are to take and how much do they really understand? Students and unemployed people are frequently the subjects of these first human studies. They are paid a relatively small fee for their services, but in view of their low income even this small amount may influence their decision to participate. Following the RCP report the government is expected to clarify these issues.

A single dose of a new drug can be given to a human volunteer provided that animal-toxicity tests have been performed for two weeks on two species of animals. But, as the human tests get longer, so the animal tests which precede them must become more detailed and include larger numbers of animals. Thus, to test a drug on a human for one to three months the drug must have been tested for six months on two species of animal.

After the so-called 'phase 1' studies on healthy human volunteers are completed the second phase of human studies begins. For the first time the drug is tested on sick patients to check that it will indeed help to relieve their symptoms. Again, only a few low doses are used initially as experience is built up. During phases '2' and '3', experience is gradually built up of the effectiveness of the drug in treating the illness for which it is designed. The ideal dose is worked out, how often it should be given and what are the common side-effects. It is only at the end of these studies that the number of patients in the study is stepped up and information about long-term use of the drug, for periods up to a year or more, is gathered. At this stage the new drug is probably on trial in several different countries and the company is assembling the final data to present to licensing authorities in countries which have specific requirements for drug testing. Since 1971, Britain has been one of these countries with specific licensing requirements. At that time the Committee on Safety of Medicines

(CSM) took over from the Committee on Safety of Drugs to assess the data from animal and clinical trials, and from this decide whether a new drug should be granted a licence for widespread use.

The Committee has nineteen members, experts in a wide range of medical specialities – from pharmacology to geriatrics, rheumatology to cardiology. They consider between 100 and 200 licence applications each year. Few are really novel drugs, and in addition to those referred to the CSM some 400 are dealt with by DHSS staff. All drugs have to pass the same animal and human tests but the most straightforward licence applications, often involving products which are variations on drugs already licensed, are assessed by the medical staff at the DHSS.

The Committee on Safety of Medicines advises the health secretary – in the guise of the Licensing Authority which grants or refuses licences. This is not unique. France, Germany, the United States of America, Canada, Australia and most western countries have their own licensing systems. Developing countries rely largely on the decisions of these countries to licence new drugs. The British Licensing Authority and its American equivalent – the Food and Drug Administration (FDA) – set the standards for other countries. But there have been criticisms. The CSM meets thirteen times a year and there is considerable communication and discussion among committee members between meetings. Their work-load is heavy and it has been suggested that there is simply too much work, both in assessing new drugs for licences and for considering problems with older drugs, for one committee to cope with.

Some observers argue that the fact that a number of drugs have slipped through the safety-net in recent years testifies to failings in the system. But members of the committee argue that a few drugs will always slip through because of the inevitable limitations on the numbers of people involved in tests before marketing. They feel they have reacted swiftly in cases where drugs have proved unsafe. A second government committee, the Committee on the Review of Medicines (CRM) is currently examining the value of all those drugs which were on the market before the Medicines Act came into force.

These drugs were granted so-called 'licences of right' to avoid the need for all of them to be re-examined immediately the Medicines Act came into force, and to give companies time to perform the trials on their drugs, as these trials had not been required before 1971. But this review has taken far longer than expected and the current deadline of 1990 is likely to be exceeded.

Monitoring Drug Side-effects

By the time a drug is licensed for general use, it will have been tested on between 1000 and 2000 people. Some subjects will have had only a single dose, others may have used it for a few weeks or months and a small proportion for as long as a year or eighteen months – not many people when you consider that within its first year on the market a new drug for a common condition such as high blood pressure or arthritis is likely to be used by some 10,000 people!

In effect, those 10,000 people are participating in, if you like, delayed clinical trials. All the legally required tests have been performed and the drug is deemed safe and effective by the authorities. But experience of the drug and its likely side-effects is still remarkably limited. The clinical trials will have picked up a severe side-effect occurring at a rate of one in 500 but a rarer problem occurring, say, in one case in 10,000 or more will only register when sufficient numbers of people have used the drug after it has come on to the market.

Unfortunately, there can be no guarantee that a new drug will not produce unforeseen serious side-effects, as Opren, Zomax, Osmosin, Flosint have proved. All these new drugs had to be withdrawn soon after they were licensed, after clinical-trial data had shown that they should be safe and effective. So what can be done to safeguard patients against new drugs whose side-effects simply have not shown up in clinical trials? One suggestion has been that drugs should be given an interim licence and introduced only slowly to the market to see whether further side-effects emerge in the months immediately after launch. But some health officials believe that such a system would be counter-productive. They feel that by introducing the drug to a large number of people as quickly as possible after launch side-effects are more likely to show up as numbers of patients using the drug mount. They fear that if a drug is used by only a small number of people initially then the incidence of side-effects would be masked and it would simply take years rather than months for the figures to accumulate.

Instead, they prefer the current system to be strengthened and improved. At present, all drugs, new and old, are subject to a system of recording drug side-effects called the yellow-card system. Each year the DHSS sends doctors throughout the country a number of yellow cards. If the doctor suspects that a patient has suffered a side-effect from a drug he is using then the doctor fills in a card and returns it to the DHSS. On it, she reports personal details of the patient – name, age, sex, the drug taken and the side-effect. The yellow cards are collected centrally by the DHSS and the information on them stored on computers. The data are regularly checked for trends in side-effects; to see whether a new drug has unforeseen effects or whether older established drugs are throwing up unusual side-effects.

In theory, such a system should be the answer. Yet only 12,000 reports of adverse reactions arrive at the DHSS from doctors and dentists each year. That means that on average a GP fills in a yellow card once every two years, and yet she has, on average, 2000 patients receiving 12,000 prescriptions each year. It is hard to imagine that only one patient reports a reaction to her out of 24,000 prescriptions which she considers important enough to report to the CSM.

The DHSS agrees. It reckons that under-reporting of side-effects is occurring on a massive scale and that doctors are reporting perhaps one in twenty of the reactions which should be reported. So obvious were the shortfalls in the current yellow-card system that in 1983 the CSM produced a report with no less than twenty-nine recommendations for improving the system. It pressed for urgent research to find out why doctors fail to report adverse reactions and what steps could be taken to encourage them to do so. It said that doctors should be trained, at medical school, to recognize and report side-effects at the earliest possible time, and that there should be more feedback to doctors about adverse reactions, so that they would feel part of a team rather than acting in isolation.

At present the DHSS issues an occasional newsletter entitled 'Current Problems' which informs doctors of any trends in side-effects so that they may be particularly aware of them. The CSM working-party recommended that this should appear more frequently and be circulated to doctors more quickly. The working-party ruled out offering a financial inducement to doctors to report more adverse reactions and it also felt that reporting should not be made a statutory requirement. So what progress has been made since the 1983 report?

The DHSS is still considering how to act on many of the CSM's recommendations. It has set up a pilot study of a new computerized system of yellow cards. Instead of a doctor physically filling in the form and sending it by post to the DHSS, 400 chosen GPs are testing this computerized scheme. They call up the DHSS through their computer terminal and a blank 'yellow card' appears on their screen. They then fill in the details of the patient and the drugs taken and 'send' the information direct to the DHSS computer.

This has several advantages over the current postal system. It is quicker and requires less effort on the part of the GP. In addition, she can get immediate feedback about other reports of the same or similar side-effects, their incidence and importance. From the DHSS point of view it is possible to get fast accurate information and the 'yellow card' does not disappear from the doctor's screen until it is completed. So there is no risk of getting half-filled cards with important details about drug dosage or the patient's age and sex missed out as can occur with the postal yellow cards.

A growing number of doctors in the country have computers. So the idea of a national network of computerized adverse-reaction reporting is not as unlikely as it would have been only a few years ago. Even so, it will not be cheap and the likelihood of it spreading immediately to all 30,000 GPs in the country overnight is small.

Schemes other than the yellow-card reporting system are in operation in other areas. One of the best-established of these is the 'prescription event monitoring system', run from the Drug Surveillance Unit (DSU) at Southampton. This examines the reactions of patients taking relatively new drugs. Forms are sent to GPs known to be prescribing the drug being studied and they record their experiences with it. The advantage of the system is that doctors are not asked to judge whether reactions experienced by their patients are related to the drug they are taking. Instead they are asked to record anything in the patient's notes which could be classed as an 'event'. This could be anything from a headache to a broken leg. The object of this is to rule out bias. The doctor may feel that the broken leg is totally unrelated. But if the Southampton centre finds that there is a relatively high incidence of broken legs in patients taking the drug there might be some suggestion that it is affecting patients' balance and is worth further investigation to check just how the fractures occurred.

Over 100,000 reports on ten drugs were collected and analysed in the first two years after the centre was set up in 1982. And in contrast to the yellow-card system, the Southampton unit has achieved a remarkably good response from GPs with its more personal approach to collecting adverse-reaction data. Overall, almost two thirds of doctors have returned forms to the unit.

So, clearly doctors can cooperate on drug monitoring given the right approach. The major drawback of the Southampton scheme is the time and cost of sending out and analysing the event forms. Only three or four drugs can be monitored at any one time and, because the system gets responses on 10–15,000 patients in each of its drug assessments, side-effects which occur more rarely than this will simply not be detected by the system.

Because of its infinite capacity for continuing to monitor patients the yellow-card system can pick up these rare side-effects – provided doctors report them.

But if doctors cannot or will not return yellow cards to the DHSS, who will? Hospital pharmacists fill in yellow cards and get doctors to sign them where they are aware that an adverse reaction has occurred. And when the local pharmacist working in the high-street chemist's has a good relationship with his GP he may be able to warn her of side-effects of drugs which come to his attention.

For example, patients frequently go to their pharmacist to buy drugs to treat symptoms caused by drugs which have been pre-scribed by their doctor. They may get indigestion from their anti-arthritis drugs, or constipation from a pain-killer. If this is a well-recognized side-effect of an established drug then there is probably no need to report it. But, if it is an unusual side-effect or the patient is taking a brand-new drug, the pharmacist is in an ideal position to question the patient about the problem and report the side-effect as a suspected result of the drug.

One method, which has been studied by doctors and pharmacists, would be for the pharmacist to fill in a yellow card and send it to the GP to sign. In this way the GP would be aware of what his patient was suffering as a result of the drug and would take the final decision on whether to report the reaction.

However, some pharmacists believe that they should be able to return yellow cards direct to the DHSS. There is considerable professional rivalry between doctors and pharmacists, which in some cases reaches such a pitch that doctors even resent pharmacists phoning to query possible mistakes on prescriptions. The reverse can also happen since many pharmacists feel they are better trained on drug usage than doctors and are critical of the way in which their local GPs prescribe. Suffice it to say that the bad feeling which exists between many pharmacists and GPs has made it difficult to devise a system of adverse-reaction reporting which would include the pharmacist, without upsetting the GP.

An even more outraged response is given to those who suggest that patients themselves could report their side-effects to the DHSS. Those working at the Department argue that they would be deluged by inaccurate or irrelevant reports of everything from ingrowing toe-nails to heart attacks apparently related to drugs.

Already, the DHSS has tried to impress on doctors that they should not send in reports of well-known side-effects associated with long-established drugs. Everyone knows, for example, that you can get indigestion from aspirin-like drugs and the DHSS does not want to know about minor effects from old drugs. They are much more interested in reactions, however trivial, from new drugs. Indigestion may be a trivial side-effect but if it occurs in 100 per cent of patients taking a new anti-arthritic drug this may be considered unacceptable in view of the fact that other similar drugs cause a much lower incidence of the same problem.

By discouraging doctors from reporting established side-effects however, the authorities may give the impression that they are not interested in side-effects which already appear on the data-sheets of relatively new drugs. For example, the photosensitivity reactions which occurred with the anti-arthritic drug Opren were recognized from the start. But their frequency and severity were much greater than originally thought. This clearly emphasizes the importance of reporting effects with new drugs where little experience has been built up during clinical trials.

Clearly, if doctors find it hard to distinguish between trivial and serious side-effects, patients would find it even more difficult. But, since it is we, the consumers/patients, who experience those side-effects, we are in the best position to explain what they are like and how bad they are. Several organizations including the Patients Liaison Group of the Royal College of General Practitioners and the Patients Association are now pressing for us, the consumers, to be allowed to report our side-effects direct to the DHSS or to some other collecting house.

In the meantime, we must rely on our doctor to report unusual or worrying side-effects. But how can we help? Everyone has experienced the patronizing smile and verbal 'pat on the head' from the doctor when they describe a problem which they think may be related to a drug. But we may well contribute to this reaction by being too vague about these symptoms. Merely saying 'I feel funny' or 'I don't feel right when I get up in the morning' is clearly not enough.

If you notice some effect which you have not previously experienced before starting to take a new drug, keep a record of when it happens. Note down the time of day you got the dizzy spell, headache or other symptom. Try and remember if you ate or drank at the same time or soon after taking the drug and what else you were doing at the time it occurred. In isolation a bad headache appearing mid-afternoon seems to be unrelated to drugs or food. But if it occurs regularly at the same time or following the same food or activity there may be some explanation for the pattern and you may be able to remove the trigger which is making the symptoms worse.

If you record these events, then when you present the problem to the doctor you have much more specific information on which she can act. She may have forgotten to mention a well-known side-effect or interaction of your drug with some other drug or food, in which case she can offer advice and set your mind at rest. Alternatively, the side-effect may be sufficiently severe for you to have to stop taking the drug.

It is extremely hard to question a doctor's judgement at the best of times and virtually impossible from a position of ignorance. A busy surgery and a queue of patients in the waiting-room do not encourage patients to discuss their theories on side-effects. There must be only a few people who, having got their GP grudgingly to admit that there may be something in their curious headaches or rashes, will suggest to their doctor that she ought to fill in a yellow card and inform the DHSS.

The Patients Association collects information about side-effects when patients write in with specific problems, as does the newer College of Health. So, if you feel strongly about your side-effect and feel that it is being ignored, that might be one outlet for your information. But neither organization has the scope to act as a central collecting house.

Compensation

There are no recorded cases in Britain of patients who have successfully sued drug companies over death, disability or injury caused by a drug; in fact, there is no record of any such case ever having come to court. Thousands of cases have come to court in litigation-conscious America and other countries have seen their share of celebrated cases against drug companies whose drugs have caused injury or disability.

Does this mean that the UK is a remarkable oasis where drug accidents never happen and where patients never suffer serious side-effects? Clearly not. The charity, Action for the Victims of Medical Accidents (AVMA) has about 100 cases on record of patients who want to sue drug companies over alleged drug injuries, the Opren Action group has another 1000, and the Association of Parents of Vaccine Damaged Children has 350.

The difference between Britain and many other western countries is that here patients must prove negligence in order to receive compensation for drug injuries. Elsewhere, patients need only show that the drug caused the alleged side-effects. This in itself is no easy target but provided that sufficient international experts agree that the injuries are unlikely to be due to chance or some other factor, the patient stands a good chance of getting compensation.

Frequently even the medical experts cannot agree about cause and effect. Some of the most difficult cases revolve around side-effects or disabilities alleged to have been caused by a drug but which can also occur as a natural development of the disease which is being treated. Equally, it is difficult to prove cause and effect if the side-effect appears to be unique and has never been seen in any patient before or since; it would seem then that it could be coincidence, which has resulted in the patient suffering the effect at the same time as taking the drug.

A number of malformations in new-born babies have been attributed to drugs taken in pregnancy. As already mentioned, it is advisable to avoid all drugs during pregnancy but this may not always be possible. Roughly 2 per cent of all babies are born with some lesser or greater degree of abnormality – by chance. This may be as minor as a hare-lip or as major as half a heart or both arms missing. Even when there is clear-cut evidence that a drug was taken at just that stage of pregnancy, when the deformity could have occurred, it may be hard to prove that it was the drug which was at fault and not mere chance. Only in cases where a group of babies are born with a specific and unusual group of abnormalities – as in the case of babies whose mothers took thalidomide – does it become more straightforward to attribute the abnormalities to the drug.

Given that it is difficult to prove even cause and effect for drug-induced injuries, consider how much harder it is if the patient has to prove that the company was, in addition, negligent in testing or developing the drug or in warning patients of likely side-effects.

Drug companies are no more equipped with crystal balls than the rest of us. They may, in good faith, research and develop a new drug, test it to all the standards laid down by the D H S S, get it licensed and then, five years later, discover an unforeseen and dangerous side-effect which simply did not appear frequently enough for it to be picked up during drug tests on limited numbers of patients. Were they then negligent or just unlucky? But how much more unlucky is the hapless patient who also in good faith took the drug, followed the instructions and finished up with a major disability which will prevent him working and leading a normal life. Should he not get some form of compensation to make up for his loss of wage-earning, to provide him with aids to make daily living easier and to go some way to repair the damage to his life?

In 1978, the Royal Commission on Civil Liability and Compensation (the Pearson Commission, named after its chairman) recommended that the law be changed so that manufacturers could be held strictly liable for any damage caused to consumers by their products. The recommendation included drugs. At around the same time the Commission of the EEC proposed new legislation to apply to all member countries broadly along the lines recommended by Pearson. Things move slowly at the EEC and the directive on product liability (as it has become known) spent nearly ten years shuffling between EEC bureaucrats before it was finally agreed in 1985. Even so, member countries have three years in which to act on it. The situation at present is that France has strict liability and so do certain parts of the United States. Sweden and New Zealand have compensation funds for victims of medical and drug accidents. West Germany, Luxemburg and Belgium all have some form of compensation.

British lawyers, however, are still stuck with having to prove negligence against any company whose products are alleged to have been defective. Is this fair? Those who are against the introduction of strict liability in Britain argue that such a system leads to the practice of defensive medicine by doctors, which is against the interests of the patient. They point to the massive awards made against doctors, hospitals and drug companies in the United States and allege that things have reached a sorry state when you work by the motto 'if it moves, sue it'.

Those who take this view believe that drug companies will not be prepared to spend the enormous amounts of money required to develop a new drug if they could be sued for millions of pounds over side-effects they had no way of foreseeing. Neither drug companies nor doctors who have to compensate patients do so out of their own pockets. They are covered by insurance schemes which pay up if their clients are successfully sued. Not surprisingly the companies which run such schemes protect themselves by inserting clauses insisting that doctors and drug companies take steps to 'cover their backs'. For example, many American doctors when diagnosing an illness perform numerous unnecessary tests just to be on the safe side. Then if they are sued they can say that they did everything possible to rule out other diseases. Similarly they may operate more frequently than in this country to protect themselves against claims from patients. They must be able to defend themselves in court by saying that every possible check and safety measure was used to ensure their patient's safety – hence the claims of 'defensive medicine'.

If defensive medicine were to be practised routinely there is little doubt that it would be the patients who suffered in the long term. Treatment would be delayed while every possible check was made and surgery or some other form of treatment might be performed 'just in case' rather than because it was really needed. This would increase waiting-lists and costs. Insurance premiums for companies to protect them against drug accidents are constantly increasing, even without the introduction of strict liability. Inevitably, this increase in premiums is passed on eventually to the patients through increasingly expensive drugs and health services.

But should the risk of defensive medicine rule out the introduction of an effective compensation scheme for people who, through no fault of their own, or the manufacturer of the drug, are damaged by their medicines? A compromise could be set up along the lines of the 'no fault' schemes in effect in Sweden and New Zealand. These are run by the state and patients who prove cause and effect of damage from their drugs are compensated out of a central fund. Where does the money for this come from? It has been suggested that the drug industry itself should be responsible for funding such a scheme and the British industry, while in favour of a central fund, believes that the money should come out of the government's pocket.

Any patient who felt he had been damaged by a drug could apply for compensation from such a fund. He would not have to prove negligence and, provided that the tribunal – composed of medical and lay representatives – were satisfied that the balance was in favour of the injury being attributed to the drug, he would receive immediate compensation from the fund. If there were grounds to believe that the drug company had, in addition, been negligent, the case could be referred through the courts and the company would have to reimburse the compensation fund.

The crucial point, however, would be that there would be no delay in the patient getting compensation if his case was proven. Patients currently trying to sue the manufacturers of Opren have already been told by their lawyers that their cases may not come to court in their lifetime and it will probably be their children who pick up any compensation if their case is proven. Few people, faced with the prospect of years of legal wrangling and mounting bills from solicitors with no guarantee of success at the end of the day, will be prepared to stake all in an attempt to get compensation for their injuries. Restrictions on the granting of legal aid for such cases have made it almost impossible for patients to get financial help to continue their case. And experience in the last year with Opren has shown that foreign courts are unhappy to hear cases referring to British patients even when the company being sued is based overseas.

Lawyers specializing in this type of case have for some time been pressing for a change in the way they are paid, bringing them in line with the system practised in America and making it easier for clients to pursue their claims without having to find enormous sums of money.

In America lawyers are paid a set proportion of the compensation granted by the courts – generally 10 per cent. This is taken into consideration by judges when granting compensation, so that clients are not unduly out of pocket. If the case fails then the lawyer gets nothing. This means that it is strongly in the lawyer's interests to win the case, equally it will discourage him from taking on a case with a very poor chance of success. In principle the introduction of such a scheme would appear to make good sense but the concept was set back in 1984 by the sight of dozens of American lawyers flying into India in the aftermath of the Bhopal disaster and signing up victims of the gas explosion in the sure knowledge of getting their 10 per cent of the vast claim put in on victims' behalfs.

Clearly, if such a percentage system were to be implemented in the United Kingdom, it would need careful monitoring to ensure that lawyers were not taking advantage of their clients. But it would ensure that patients did not have to face bankruptcy in order to stand any chance of getting compensation for their injuries.

CHAPTER 5

Successes and Failures of Modern Drugs

How many drugs can you remember by name? Aspirin, penicillin, Valium . . . If you are a diabetic you probably mentioned insulin; if you have high blood pressure you probably thought of Inderal; and if you suffer from arthritis you probably added Brufen to your list. But the rest of us, who are lucky enough not to have any chronic illness, would probably be hard pressed to come up with more than a handful of drugs other than cough and cold remedies.

Over 17,000 drug products are licensed for use in Britain. That figure is rather misleading since some drugs have three or four licences covering different doses and formulations – tablets, liquid and injections, for example. It also includes a number of drugs which are no longer marketed but manufacturers have held on to their licences for a rainy day. Less than a third of all these drugs are listed in the doctors' handbook, the *British National Formulary*, which ranks drugs according to cost and effectiveness. And, realistically, doctors write most of their prescriptions from perhaps 300 drugs which they have used for many years and feel at home with. Periodically, they may be sufficiently impressed with a new drug that they tack it on to their list and perhaps jettison one or two outdated products.

Yet for all these armies of drugs which are available there are still vast gaps; diseases for which there are few, if any, effective drugs and conditions which are poorly understood by the medical profession. Unfortunately, drug companies cannot produce breakthroughs to order. Aspirin, penicillin, insulin and, more recently, beta-blockers, contraceptive pills and anti-ulcer drugs have all been important advances. Not surprisingly, however, having spent an average of £25 million developing a new drug, a company is loath to throw it down the laboratory sink just because it is not the best thing since penicillin. The market for heart drugs is worth over £100 million a year in the United Kingdom alone; another £32 million is spent on tranquillizers and a further £50 million on penicillins. Putting aside the manufacturing costs, a drug which captured 10 per cent of such a market would recoup its research and development costs in five years. Even taking into consideration the overheads and costs of ingredients, a company with a new drug in one of the big therapeutic areas is quickly making a profit. So, although the big breakthroughs collar the largest share of the prize money, the also-rans, or 'me toos', as they are called in drug circles, can also give a healthy return for an each-way bet.

There is a growing feeling, however, that a new drug should not only have to be proved safe and effective, it should also have to prove that it has real advantages over similar drugs already on the market – that it is really needed. By setting up a committee to judge the relative merits of new drugs vying for a place on the limited list of drugs already drawn for some types of illness, the government has put in motion the beginnings of a system to assess need as well as safety and effectiveness. Some countries, such as Norway, have already taken this path and now insist that manufacturers of new drugs prove that their product is really necessary for an illness not catered for by other drugs already available. The drug industry argues that it needs the profits from its 'me toos' to fund research designed to discover the real breakthroughs. The problem lies in striking a balance between too few breakthroughs and too many 'me toos'.

Some 'me toos' are undoubtedly needed, not just to boost drug company research funds – and profits – but because people do respond differently to drugs which, to the pharmacologists, are almost identical. Nowhere is this more true than in the field of arthritis where a patient can fail to respond to ten drugs from the same family of chemicals but find that the eleventh drug works perfectly. But where should the line be drawn? Should each new drug have an advantage either in increased potency or fewer side-effects, than similar products already on the market? Should firms be forced to concentrate on finding that elusive cure for cancer or heart disease rather than turning out dozens of lucrative but scarcely advantageous 'me toos'? Or would this kill the golden goose and stop it from laying those occasional, life-saving golden eggs?

The Golden Eggs

To look at all the golden eggs which have been laid by the drug industry – not to mention the feathers in the nest – would take a book in itself. One area of medicine which best exemplifies the successes and failures of modern drugs and has had more than its fair share of good and bad eggs is pain. Here have been some of the greatest success stories and the most miserable failures.

Pain is a symptom which generally indicates something is wrong. Cancer, heart disease, spine and limb diseases, and stomach ulcers can all have pain as their main symptom; so does a simple headache which is nothing more than that – an indicator of neither head injury nor brain tumour, nor a response to environmental stress. Pain unites us all. Everyone has at some time experienced pain – short and sharp, dull, nagging, long and intense. It may respond to a simple aspirin or it may require morphine. It may mean major surgery or a radical change in diet or lifestyle. It gets to us all.

Aspirin

There are people still alive who can remember a world without aspirin; although it had been available as willowbark since 1780, it was first synthesized in 1853 but did not become widely available until the turn of the century. What did people do before it arrived? With a few exceptions, they relied on herbal remedies for their ailments right up till the twentieth century, and in some cases, well into it.

It was not until about eighty years after aspirin was synthesized that scientists began to understand how it actually works. They discovered that it blocks the production of a group of chemicals called prostaglandins which have the delightful task of causing pain, inflammation and fever; the body's own killjoys. As more was known of how aspirin worked, the dangerous side of its nature emerged more clearly. The risk of stomach irritation and bleeding is now so well known that it is said that if aspirin had been discovered after the present drug-testing requirements were set up it would never have got a licence. Instead, aspirin is so much a part of our culture that it could not possibly be banned. But those who suffer from stomach problems are increasingly warned that they should use paracetamol and even those with healthy stomachs are turning to alternative pain-killers.

Aspirin has many other uses in addition to relieving pain. Many people take it in very small doses to prevent heart attacks, other circulation problems, and even cataracts. From aspirin has come a vast army of pain-killing drugs. Related to them is an equally large number of drugs based on propionic acid – a chemical which also blocks prostaglandin production. And these too are important pain-killers and anti-inflammatory drugs especially in the field of arthritis. All have very similar effects, some with a few more, others with a few less side-effects. Some are better at relieving pain, others at reducing swelling in patients with inflamed joints or muscles.

But all the aspirin-like drugs have the limitation that while they can relieve some of the symptoms of arthritis, and back and muscle injuries, they cannot get at the underlying mechanisms which are at fault. It is a bit like putting oil in a car with a leaky oil system. It prevents the engine from seizing up through lack of lubrication but it does not solve the problem of the leak. You can get new parts for cars but it is not always possible to replace worn-out hips, knees and backbones. The most which orthodox medicine frequently has to offer is a patching-up job and the relief of painful symptoms. Small wonder that patients are going elsewhere in search of help for their bad backs and stiff joints.

A recent survey showed that over a million people are spending around £40 million on visits to osteopaths, acupuncturists and other alternative therapists mainly because orthodox medicine cannot help them. And the number is growing at a rate of 150,000 people a year. Osteopaths and acupuncturists, both of whom concentrate on conditions whose main symptom is pain, are two of the groups most frequently consulted. It seems that people are no longer content to trundle from specialist to specialist operating within the health service only to be told there is nothing obviously wrong with their back, their shoulder, their knee and they will simply have to go home and rest the offending part. Even when the evidence of disease is only too obvious – such as in the arthritic joint – orthodox medicine may have nothing to offer.

This is not to say that the osteopaths, the chiropractors, the acupuncturists, herbalists and homeopaths have miracle cures but many people who have exhausted all that conventional medicine has to offer feel that they have nothing to lose. But what are they getting instead? What happens to the patient with back pain who seeks help from alternative practitioners? What can he expect? What will he pay and, most important of all, will it work?

Joan was getting so much pain in her chest and shortness of breath that her doctor referred her to the hospital for tests. It was found that some of the arteries to her heart were blocked and she was asked if she would consider a bypass operation.

'I didn't want surgery like that and my son suggested I try a homeopathic doctor to see if he could get rid of the chest pain. I take these powders now and they seem to work very well. I have bad days but I find I can walk to the top of a nearby hill without any trouble, where once I wouldn't have dreamt of it.'

Kathleen has tried everything for her arthritis. The trouble started in her neck but now the disease has spread to her arms and legs, hands and feet. Once a very active person, Kathleen can hardly get to the shops or do her housework. She has bought a food processor because the pain of standing and mixing the flour prevented her from making pastry.

'I have tried so many different drugs. Sometimes they work for a while, but it seems that I always end up with side-effects. Some of them upset my stomach, some gave me headaches, one even sent me deaf until I adjusted the dose,' said Kathleen.

Now she relies on paracetamol alone for when the pain is at its worst, and the rest of the time has to put up with it. She's also tried heat treatment, which did not have much effect.

'I just wish they could discover something which would relieve the pain without the side-effects: something you could just take when you were in pain rather than having to take all the time.'

As a child Hazel had polio. She made a full recovery but wonders whether the back problems she has experienced in later life are related to her earlier illness. About eight years ago she slipped a disc in her back while doing some gardening. Bed-rest and pain-killing drugs helped improve her condition and, a little uncertainly, Hazel went back to work as a cook.

Standing up all day aggravated the back problem and Hazel went from doctor to doctor for help. Eventually her back became so bad that she had to give up work and doctors diagnosed arthritis in her spine.

Now Hazel sees an osteopath who, she believes, has dramatically improved her back. She still walks with a limp and finds it hard to do her housework and get the shopping, but things are much better than they were.

'Once my back has settled down after each treatment I get far less pain than before. This goes on for several days and then I know I am getting near to needing another session of osteopathy. It has made a big difference to me though; I need fewer pain-killing drugs and I can get about much more easily.'

Going to an Osteopath

Up to thirty million working days are thought to be lost each year through back pain. Treatment for the vast majority of patients centres on lying flat on their back and taking analgesics until the pain disappears and they can get up and about again. But, as thousands of people can testify, once a weak back, always a weak back. Sometimes the problem shows up on an X-ray and gets a medical name; other times there is no specific diagnosis and the patient goes away with 'lumbago' – a simple name for 'we don't know what's wrong' or 'we can't really help'.

A growing number of people with back pain are not content with their vague diagnosis, pain-killers and bed-rest, and go in search of treatment which will not just relieve their painful symptoms but will attempt to correct the underlying disorder. The osteopath, like most alternative therapists, takes a much more holistic approach to injury and disease than the medical profession. He does not see the back in isolation from the rest of the body and he tries to relate symptoms in one part of the body to disorders elsewhere. A leading osteopath summed up the difference between the medical approach and his own in a recent case involving a doctor turned patient.

The doctor went to the osteopath with a painful knee which could barely take any weight. His medical colleagues could find nothing wrong with the knee and had little to offer in the way of treatment. When the osteopath looked at it he too could neither see nor feel anything wrong. Then he turned to his patient's back – had there ever been any trouble in the lower part of the spine? Yes, in the past, said the doctor, but not recently. A careful examination did reveal an abnormality in the spine which was putting pressure on the knee. It was easily corrected and the knee soon returned to normal.

At the other end of the body, someone complaining of headaches or pain in their neck and shoulders may well have some minor abnormality in their back which is putting pressure on other tissues. And an osteopath would be as likely to examine their vertebrae as their neck or shoulders.

In order to be able to relate apparently unrelated ailments the osteopath must have a knowledge of anatomy and physiology at least as good as that of the doctor. He must know how muscles and nerves in one part of the body interact with those in another. This is why it is essential that the osteopath is properly trained. Two of the London-based schools of osteopathy, the British School of Osteopathy and the London School of Osteopathy, put their students through four- and five-year trainings consisting of a mixture of theoretical study and practical classes. Initially, students practise on each other and then they are taken on as trainees to experienced osteopaths, rather like GPs in the NHS, to treat real patients.

Inevitably, unqualified people do set themselves up in practice and it is frequently they who give the rest of the profession a bad name. If you are trying to find a properly trained osteopath you can contact the Institute for Complementary Medicine in London which keeps lists of qualified practitioners in different areas or you can check whether an osteopath is on the register of osteopaths which entitles him to put MRO after his name and basic qualification. Osteopathy is rarely available on the NHS. Some GPs do practise osteopathy or will refer patients to local osteopaths who charge around £10 per session.

An interesting experiment is currently under way at Derby Royal Infirmary where a trained osteopath is contracted to the health authority to provide osteopathy on the NHS, half a day a week. Orthopaedic surgeons at the hospital pass a motley collection of back problems to this osteopath, but in general they are problem patients for whom orthodox medicine has nothing to offer. A research project to measure just how effective osteopathy is in correcting spinal problems is continuing alongside the NHS work. Patients are wired up to electrodes which feed information into a computer which can assess just what effect the osteopath is having on the re-adjustment of their spine. This is one of the first experiments to try and measure quantitatively just what osteopathy does. Qualitative reactions from patients – that they feel better or worse after treatment – are not enough for science. It must have precise measurements on paper of benefit. Alternative therapists have been criticized in the past for failing to submit their techniques to scientific analysis and for relying too much on anecdotal reports of the success of their treatments.

Alternative therapies do not lend themselves easily to scientific analysis. It is relatively easy to compare the effectiveness of a new drug against placebo, without doctor or patient knowing who is on active treatment and who is taking the placebo. The tablets look the same. But it is rather more difficult to find a placebo for osteopathy; patients tend to know whether their back is being manipulated or not. It would not be difficult, however, to compare the long-term effects of osteopathy with, say, bed-rest and analgesics in patients with the same kind of back problem. And at last, alternative therapists are taking up the challenge from their orthodox colleagues to carry out proper research. But in the meantime, alternative therapists not unreasonably point out that patients would not keep coming back to them, paying for treatment, if they did not feel some benefit.

Although most people only go to an osteopath when they have something wrong with their back, many therapists believe that people should have regular back checks just as they would have their teeth inspected every six months or so. They argue that the human spine is not geared for the punishing routine we put it through and that although only a proportion of people have bad backs we should all have checks to ensure that everything is in working order.

Osteopaths also believe they have a lot to offer arthritis sufferers. They do not claim to cure the disease once the degenerative processes are well advanced but they believe that by stretching and rotating the joints when the disease is still in its early stages they can keep the patient mobile and postpone the day when they will need a joint replacement or become housebound. Arthritis in one form or another is thought to afflict over six million people in the United Kingdom and as the number of elderly people continues to increase, the figures for arthritis victims can only rise too. Drugs may help to relieve the pain and a few have some effect on the disease. But anything which can help to slow the degenerative processes must have some value.

Acupuncture in Pain Relief

A mere 2000 or so years since its first recorded use, acupuncture has gained a degree of acceptance amongst western doctors which other therapists can only dream of. Even the most sceptical doctors are now admitting that 'there's something in acupuncture'. Many NHS pain clinics offer some form of nerve stimulation – whether by acupuncture needles or electrodes – in their range of treatments. Some 600 doctors have joined the British Medical Acupuncture Society, and use the technique to a greater or lesser degree in their everyday work. Even the working party of the British Medical Association which has been doing its own analysis of alternative therapies is known to favour acupuncture when other therapies have received short shrift.

But, having taken acupuncture into the fold, many doctors now believe that they are the only people sufficiently knowledgeable of the anatomy and physiology of the body, who should be let loose with the needles. True, there are many people practising acupuncture who do not know what they are doing. But those trained in traditional Chinese acupuncture believe that their three years of study and practical experience are sufficient to enable them to practise competently. In addition, they feel that many doctors who have taken up acupuncture have rather missed the point because they do not go along with the whole Chinese medical philosophy of maintaining a balance of energy within the body. Doctors may stimulate acupuncture points to great effect but without an acceptance of the underlying philosophy of energy flow through the body they cannot achieve maximum benefit, say the traditional acupuncturists.

It is a bit like playing a fruit machine. A couple of oranges or apples can win you small prizes but you have got to line up all three pictures to get the jackpot.

In the last twenty years, two discoveries in the field of pain control have put scientifically based theory behind the obvious practical success of acupuncture and contributed to its greater acceptance by the medical profession. First, in the mid-Sixties, came the discovery that there appear to be two types of nerve fibre which can transmit pain. One appears to transmit pain itself, while the other is responsible for enabling us to be aware of touch – in effect, pain, but much more dilute. The theory was that as long as stimulation of the 'touch' fibres exceeds that of the 'pain' fibres we are not in pain. And direct stimulation of the touch fibres, by acupuncture, for example, could be at the root of some methods of pain relief. Subsequent research has shown that the mechanism is not quite as simple as that but it is believed to play some part in acupuncture.

Ten years on from this so-called pain-gating theory came the discovery of the body's natural pain-killers, the endorphins. Acupuncture got another boost when it was found that nerve stimulation triggered release of these endorphins and also of other nerve transmitters involved in passing on pain. Now that science had lent credence to acupuncture, doctors came up with their own methods of nerve stimulation, but based on traditional tried-and-tested acupuncture points.

Traditional acupuncturists are quite happy with the new-found scientific theories; after all, they had always said that acupuncture triggered hormones and other chemicals in the body – they were just a bit less specific about which ones were involved. But they are sticking with their theory, established over millennia, rather than decades, that acupuncture points are linked by meridians along which flows the vital energy. Interrupt that path, either by stimulation or inhibition of acupuncture points, and you will alter the state of the organs and tissues which lie along it.

Whatever their differences over the theory of acupuncture, doctors and traditional acupuncturists are becoming increasingly united over the conditions where the technique works best. As with osteopathy, people tended initially to take to alternative therapists painful conditions that had not responded to western medicine. Thus acupuncturists see a high proportion of people with backache, arthritis, muscle and soft tissue pain. And some acupuncturists work with osteopaths to relieve bone and joint pains. The osteopathy releases the muscle spasm and readjusts discs and vertebrae while the acupuncture relieves pain and helps to reduce inflammation.

Like osteopaths, acupuncturists do not profess to cure arthritis. Nothing short of a hip or knee replacement is going to get the chair-bound arthritic moving about again, and even that may not be totally successful. But acupuncturists believe that by reducing pain and inflammation in the joints they can help to keep the patient mobile, thus postponing joint degeneration and the need for surgery.

Other painful conditions frequently treated to great effect by acupuncture include migraine and dysmenorrhoea – period pain. Some acupuncturists claim 80–90 per cent success rates in the treatment of migraine. People suffering two or three migraines a week have shown dramatic improvement following courses of acupuncture. And women afflicted with severe period pains, month after month, have also responded to acupuncture where drugs have failed dismally to achieve any success.

How many courses of treatment do people need? Just as people vary in their requirement for medicines, so they vary in their need for acupuncture. One leading acupuncturist claims that if he has not relieved period pains within three months, involving perhaps six treatments, then he assumes he has failed – but this does not happen often. Migraine can require anything from fifteen to fifty treatments, depending on how severe it is, and patients with arthritis may need long-term, regular acupuncture, perhaps for several years.

Acupuncturists can tell, to some extent, whether the treatment will work from the initial responses of patients. People who get some immediate relief, even if it is short-lived and lasts only a few hours, are more likely to benefit from further treatment. They are generally the ones who 'feel something' when the needles have been inserted. This should not be painful, just a sensation that something foreign has gone into their tissues. Frequently, acupuncturists wiggle the needles around once they have been inserted to find where the patient gets the most sensation. But people who feel nothing are less likely to respond in the longer term. Ideally, the patient has a series of treatments, perhaps once a week or once a fortnight if they seem to be responding, for a period of three to six months. And once their pain has been effectively relieved they will probably only need a 'top up' every six months or so.

Acupuncturists do express frustration that people expect too much too soon. Limitations on time and money prevent many people from going for acupuncture more frequently than once a fortnight or once a month. But many acupuncturists believe they would respond much more quickly if they had an intensive course of treatment with acupuncture every day or even several times a day, as occurs when the therapy is practised in China.

Chronic and regular acute pain, such as occur in arthritis and migraine, are not the only forms of pain which are widely acknowledged to respond to acupuncture. The technique has also been used to control pain in one-off events such as surgical operations and childbirth.

Most of us undergo a general anaesthetic for surgery without any problem at all. But, for some people with chronic illnesses or who are severely overweight, a general anaesthetic is dangerous. Instead they may be given a spinal injection or, if their operation is minor, a local anaesthetic. But strategically placed acupuncture needles have been used successfully as an alternative.

Many women are unhappy about the options for pain relief currently available during childbirth. Some drugs can cross the placenta and make the baby quiet and listless when it is born and others, used in epidural injections, can make it hard for the woman to push properly during labour. A good epidural knocks out only the nerves which are transmitting pain from the womb. But when the epidural is less precise, it can knock out nerves which are needed to trigger the muscles required to push the baby out. Labours where an epidural is given tend to be longer and are more likely to require a forceps delivery. They may also leave the mother frustrated that she has not really taken part in the delivery.

Acupuncture is being offered as an alternative form of pain relief during childbirth by a handful of doctors around the country. The technique does not guarantee a pain-free labour. But it is likely to take the edge off the pain while leaving the mother able to participate fully in the birth. When acupuncture is used in both anaesthesia for operations and in childbirth, the needles are generally attached to electrodes which are triggered to provide prolonged stimulation of the needles. Few acupuncturists would have the stamina to rotate their needles manually for several hours!

Good acupuncturists are still relatively thin on the ground. If you do want to try acupuncture for pain relief – or for the many other conditions such as allergies, drug addiction or infections which are claimed to respond to the technique – you have two options. Either you can try to find a medically qualified acupuncturist, possibly through the British Medical Acupuncture Society. Or you can ask the Institute for Complementary Medicine for the name of an acupuncturist practising in your area. The Institute only includes members of accepted traditional acupuncture societies on its register and these will have received full training in the technique. As a rough guide, you should be looking for people with BAc (Bachelor of Acupuncture) or Doctor of Acupuncture after their name. And you can expect to pay between £10 and £20 per session for treatment.

Stomach Ulcers

Drug treatment of pain does not always rest only on the relief of symptoms. Doctors may not be able to cure back pain or arthritis with drugs but they can cure stomach ulcers. One of the biggest success stories in conventional medicine of the last twenty years has been the discovery of drugs which do not just relieve the painful symptoms of stomach ulcers, they actually stop the overproduction of acid in the stomach which causes the ulcers in the first place.

Indigestion and stomach pain do not necessarily signify ulcers. Most people only need symptomatic relief. They take simple antacids which, as the name suggests, balance out the excess acid in the stomach. They do not stop the acid from being produced but they act in opposition to it to reduce the overall acid level in the stomach. Sometimes, this is not enough. People get ulcers either in the stomach itself or in the upper part of their intestine, leading from the stomach. The ulcer has a 'fried egg' appearance with a central pitted section surrounded by a less inflamed area. Many people live for years with their ulcers but before the advent of the new anti-ulcer drugs, the most serious ulcers had to be surgically removed rather than risk the possibility that they might rupture and cause a serious haemorrhage.

The problem with this approach was that the ulcers frequently returned and the only solution was to break the nerves to the stomach which controlled acid secretion, with the result that acid production was permanently blocked. The stomach does need some acid, apparently to keep it sterilized – that is why the acid is there – so a total block in production left the digestive processes impaired. In addition, the operation itself carried its own risks.

The stomach relies on receptors to mediate the nervous and hormonal stimulation of acid release. In the late Sixties it was found that it was possible to block these histamine receptors (called H2) in the stomach, and reduce production of acid. The group of drugs developed for the purpose were called H2-blockers and the first drug of this type was called cimetidine, brand name Tagamet. This drug revolutionized the treatment of ulcers; doctors were no longer having to treat the results of the extra acid – the pain and indigestion – they could actually reduce the amount of acid being produced.

Tagamet was not just a boon for patients with ulcers and their doctors who were able, overnight, to put away their scalpels. So successful was the product that it turned an ailing American drug company called Smith Kline into the darling of the stock-markets. The term, Tagamania, was coined on Wall Street; Smith Kline cornered a market worth several hundred millions of pounds a year and Tagamet remains the single most commonly prescribed drug in the United Kingdom today.

Some patients need only a single course of treatment to clear up their ulcers; others relapse when treatment is stopped and so they may need almost continuous treatment. Many gastric specialists have become worried that doctors are handing out Tagamet too freely, frequently before they have even checked that their patients do have stomach ulcers. They believe that H2-blockers should never be given until tests have confirmed that an ulcer is present and that there are no signs of cancer. Otherwise there is the risk that patients will feel better with the drug and a tumour may go undiagnosed until it is too late to treat it. In addition, patients do not always help themselves. Smoking aggravates stomach ulcers and can stop them from healing. Stress, too, is thought to contribute to the development of ulcers as is excessive caffeine intake. So people with ulcers should give up smoking and avoid stressful situations as well as relying on drugs to clear up their condition.

One day Frank was rushed to hospital vomiting blood. A quick look down into his stomach showed a large inflamed ulcer. The bleeding stopped and Frank was prescribed one of the new drugs which stops the stomach from producing the acid which leads to the formation of ulcers.

'It was marvellous; the pain stopped and I found I could eat many of the things I had had to stop eating because of the indigestion. I still can't drink spirits, but at least I can drink my beer.'

Frank has his own small business writing computer programs. As the business has expanded it has become increasingly stressful, and this probably contributed to the development of his ulcer. But thanks to the drugs Frank has been able to continue his work and plays cricket and squash when he gets the time.

Such was the overnight success of Tagamet that other drug companies have spent the ten years since it first came on to the market developing their own H2-blocking drugs in order to break Smith Kline's hold on the market. Glaxo was the first company to bring out a rival drug, called ranitidine, or Zantac, and this has already made steady inroads in the market. Further drugs of the same type are expected from a number of companies within the next few years.

A breakthrough on the scale of Tagamet is rare. Indeed the previous breakthrough before Tagamet could be said to be the beta-blocker, propranolol, called Inderal by its manufacturers.

Curiously, the same man, Sir James Black, was responsible for both discoveries: first the beta-blocker and then the H2-blocker. Beta-blockers also have a role in pain – this time the angina pain of diseased arteries. They are also important drugs in the management of high blood pressure and abnormal heart rhythms.

The beta-blockers had an inauspicious start. Practolol, called Eraldin by ICI, preceded Inderal but it was found to cause a series of severe side-effects affecting the eyes, abdominal and connective tissues, and it was subsequently withdrawn for all but the most severe cases of hypertension which were unresponsive to other drugs.

Inderal was first marketed in the early Sixties; today there are nine different types of beta-blocker and twenty-one branded products on the market. That does not include generic versions, nor the various formulations of the drugs. Another ten years and there will probably be almost as many H2-blockers, each with slight and often imagined advantages over each other, just as some beta-blockers have minor differences in properties to each other. The use of beta-blockers has been extended. Companies searching for untapped markets in which to slot their drugs discovered that one beta-blocker was useful in lowering the pressure in the eyes of patients with glaucoma, and people suffering from migraine also benefit from beta-blockers. Most recently, it has been found that beta-blockers given after a heart attack can reduce the risk of further attacks.

When you have a breakthrough drug you do not just sit back and watch the profits pile up; you find ways of exploiting every possible property of the drug to treat as many conditions as you can.

Are Drug Companies Doing Enough Research into New Drugs?

Seven nations account for three quarters of all the money spent on drug research around the world and Britain is one of them. The others are West Germany, the United States, France, Japan, Italy and Switzerland. Together, drug companies from these countries spent over £3 billion on research in 1982. Overall, that amounts to 8.6 per cent of turnover, though some countries spend more than others. Swiss companies, for example, spend just over 15 per cent of output on research, British companies spend around 12 per cent and, at the bottom end of the spectrum, Japan spends about six per cent of turnover on research and development. The figure for Japan is perhaps confusing since the country comes second only to the United States in the amount of money it spends on research. It is just that the Japanese are such massive producers of drugs that their research spending seems rather small in comparison. In addition, drug prices have been very high in Japan. Until recently Japanese companies tended to rely on western countries to come up with the ideas for new drugs, which they would then develop for themselves. Now, the Japanese drug industry looks set for the same kind of success it has had in the electrical and car industries for the last twenty years.

The figures look good on paper – anything with billion after it tends to sound pretty big. But critics of the industry, as was pointed out earlier, argue that too much of this money is spent on the 'me too' drugs and not enough on finding really new drugs. Industry figures show that almost 1500 new substances came on the market between 1961 and 1980. These drugs were new chemicals but the vast majority were related to products already on the market. Even so, it is interesting to look at the breakdown of these 'new' substances according to the countries in which they were developed.

Top of the league, with 353 new substances, were the United States, followed by France, West Germany, Japan, Italy and Switzerland. Just ahead of Great Britain came the entire Eastern Bloc. Russia and its allies are not known for their innovative prowess. In fact, western drug companies frequently cite the lack of competition, or need for profitability, between rival communist companies as one reason for the lack of new drugs coming out of countries which surely must have the potential for producing important new drugs. If they can get people into space, surely the Russians should be able to come up with some new heart or arthritis drugs, if not a cure for cancer.

The number of new drugs coming on to the market each year

has fallen steadily worldwide over the last twenty-five years, from over ninety new drugs per year in 1961 to only forty-eight in 1980. When a new drug is released it is not marketed all over the world. For example, in Britain we get about twenty new drugs each year. No one has yet been able to classify those drugs according to their real importance. Opinions vary and a drug which one person sees as an important advance may appear to be just another 'me too' to other people. No one doubts the major breakthroughs – the Inderals and the Tagamets – and everyone is aware of the copies which are no advance whatsoever on drugs already available. It is the drugs in between which cause so much debate. These may be marginally more effective than their predecessors or they may be especially useful in certain groups of patients – children, the elderly, those with other chronic diseases, for example. Or they may have a few less side-effects or their unwanted effects may occur slightly less often.

A good example of this is a relatively new group of drugs which lower blood pressure by blocking an important enzyme in blood-pressure control which is found in the kidney. The first drug of this type, called captopril, was effective in reducing blood pressure but it was linked to a number of cases of serious blood disorders. Lowering the dose reduced the incidence of such cases. But the second drug in this group, called enalapril, does not seem to be so likely to cause the blood problems. It may be that this is because it has been used in lower doses and longer experience will be needed to assess the relative advantages and disadvantages of the two drugs. On paper, enalapril, as the second drug of its type to come on to the market, would appear to be a 'me too'. And only a more detailed assessment of its properties shows advantages.

Such advantages do not have to come only in terms of effectiveness or side-effects. Dose may also be important, especially if the drug is likely to be taken by an elderly person or someone on several different kinds of medicine. These patients may find it hard to remember all their drugs, so if one of them only has to be taken once a day instead of three or four times this may make it sufficient of an advance to take it out of the lowest 'me too' category. Sometimes it is only quite late in the day that advantages of one drug over another come to light. New uses for old drugs tend to materialize only when the drug has been around for a few years.

The drug industry argues that if companies must prove that there is a need for their new drugs, and not just that they are safe and effective, as at present, many of the incidental advantages of new drugs will be lost. They will never get the chance to show that their particular heart drug causes less nausea or their anti-arthritic agent less indigestion. Knowing that it will be difficult to get a beta-blocker or an anti-inflammatory drug through the 'need' test they simply would not bother to research and develop it.

Will fewer 'me toos' mean more breakthroughs? If companies stop wasting their time looking for more beta-blockers will they spend more time finding a cure for cancer? Most of the major research-oriented drug companies at present expect to come up with a major new drug – possibly not a breakthrough, but definitely better than a 'me too' – once every ten years. So clearly they need a few lesser products in between to keep them in test tubes. But who is to decide when a company should put away its copying books and turn its attention to finding some really new drugs. Some of the Scandinavian countries may have taken the bold step of refusing licences to 'me toos' but then their companies are hardly renowned for discovering the break-through drugs, as the British pharmaceutical industry is only too happy to point out.

Future Drugs

Doctors may not look very fashion-conscious but fashions in medicine can change as quickly as the high-street hemline. It was only twenty years ago that doctors were taking teeth out in the belief that they were storing 'poisons' that were afflicting the rest of the body. The concept of focal sepsis – a disease caused by something in a totally different part of the body – died hard. Other fashions have also remained. Many children still have their tonsils taken out unnecessarily and a significant number of healthy appendixes are removed each year 'just to be on the safe side'. Only ten years ago women with breast cancer had not only the diseased breast removed but all the underlying muscle tissue and glands under the arm, leaving them sadly disfigured. Today, many surgeons favour the removal of only the lump, leaving the breast intact in the vast majority of cases.

In medicine a form of treatment takes hold and everyone practises it until someone shows a better way of tackling the problem or proves that the theory behind the treatment is faulty. The particular area of medicine under the microscope depends very much on its frequency in the population. In the Thirties it was tuberculosis, today it is cancer.

Fashions in drug research change too. When tuberculosis, diphtheria and pneumonia were still major killers and the sulphonamides and penicillin only recently discovered, the search was on for bigger and better antibiotics. The search is by no means over – there will always be a need for more specific and more powerful antibiotic treatment. But big changes have occurred in other areas of medicine.

The underlying clue to these changes is a basic shift in thinking, from trying to treat symptoms to attempting to get at the faults in the underlying mechanisms and correct them – thus curing rather than merely treating the disease. In order to correct these mechanisms scientists must learn more about the basic physiology of the human body. This is why the academic research that concentrates on how and why things happen rather than 'what's in it for us', is so important in pointing drug researchers in the right direction for major new discoveries.

It has been only in the last decade that scientists have begun to understand some of the chemical and immunological abnormalities which occur in allergic and degenerative disorders such as asthma and arthritis. Another ten years and this could mean that instead of treating the pain and inflammation of arthritis they will be able to stop the joint degeneration which causes those symptoms. The same goes for allergies; we already have drugs which, to some degree, prevent the onset of symptoms by stabilizing the cells which overreact to common substances in the air such as grass pollen and animal fur. But we need drugs which will work for all patients and not just for a minority.

Advances in drugs to treat hypertension are now concentrating on the faulty mechanisms of blood-pressure control which occur in each patient rather than merely lowering blood pressure. We may not ever be able to prevent heart attacks but we must be on the right track, improving diet and exercise to try and protect against attacks rather than waiting for the arteries to get clogged up and require major surgery.

Inevitably today's research is concentrating on the big killers of our time – cancer and heart disease. Conquering them will not mean the end of the line for research; there will always be new challenges for scientists. And just as they overcame tuberculosis by improving living conditions, vaccination and drugs, only to face new killers, so it will be with heart disease and cancer.

Cancer

The ultimate solution to cancer will be prevention rather than cure. Only when scientists discover exactly how external environmental factors, such as nicotine, chemicals, stress and personality interact with basic genetic susceptibility to the disease will they be able to protect those most at risk. Never have the signs been more optimistic. Advances in the technology which enables scientists to look at what goes wrong in cancer are enabling them to devise methods of reversing or preventing these changes.

What makes a normally growing piece of tissue suddenly go out of control, causing its cells to multiply at such a furious rate that it destroys all in its path? Recent discoveries have shown that some people have some of the same genes as viruses which cause cancer. How have these people incorporated those genes into their cells over generations and is there any way to turn them off?

At present, cancer specialists have to rely on only a handful of drugs for the treatment of the disease. So research is concentrating not only on totally new lines of therapy such as preventing the cells from becoming cancerous but also on new drugs to kill the tumours more selectively and with fewer side-effects than currently used drugs.

Heart Disease

The need for drugs to reduce blood pressure is not likely to go away. But the new breed of drugs – those which try to correct defects in the kidney and in the arterial walls – look set to take over from traditional forms of therapy which act in the heart or the blood vessels to make them compensate for the defect rather than correcting it.

Drugs which also look set to make a significant impact on the market for heart and circulatory conditions are those which actually dissolve the blood clots that block arteries to the heart and eventually result in heart attacks. The newest drugs are aimed either at breaking up the clots safely and effectively or at repairing damage to the walls of the arteries and preventing blood clots from attaching themselves there in the first place.

Arthritis

The full story of how arthritis occurs has yet to be unravelled. But it seems that overproduction of natural chemicals in the joints causes the body's defence cells to rush in and try and clear up the damage. Instead of doing this, however, they add to the vicious circle already set up and exacerbate the inflammation and degeneration. New drugs will try either to stop the chemicals from getting out of control in the first place or to prevent the immune cells from overreacting in such a catastrophic way to the initial irritation.

Simply producing more 'me toos' similar to the fifty or so anti-inflammatory products already on the market will no longer be enough. The writing is on the wall for such drugs and they are potential candidates for the government's limited list of drugs, if it is extended. In the wake of the disasters with Opren, Osmosin and Flosint – all new anti-arthritic drugs – the government is likely to insist that new drugs of this class have real and not just imagined advantages over rival products.

Merely having no more side-effects than anti-arthritic drugs which have been on the market ten or twenty years will no longer be enough to guarantee a licence. And even long-established products cannot be guaranteed a continued market, as the recent case of the butazone group of drugs showed.

This group of drugs, of which phenylbutazone and oxy-phenbutazone are the best known, had been used to relieve symptoms of arthritis for over twenty years before it was decided in 1984 that the incidence of a rare bone marrow disorder called aplastic anaemia, albeit low, was too high in relation to the effectiveness of the drugs. So one was banned altogether and another severely restricted. They had been considered worthwhile when they were first used in the past but the advent of newer, more effective drugs with fewer side-effects has made them outdated.

Contraception

With a significant number of women now in need of safer, more effective contraception for physical reasons, and others unhappy about 'messing up their hormones', scientists have started to look again at totally new methods of contraception, and to rethink the older methods.

One option has been to look at hormones produced in the brain which have overall control over the oestrogen and progesterone released from the ovaries. By upsetting the production of these brain hormones, the release of the egg can be impaired without a woman having to take large doses of synthetic oestrogen and progestogen each day. This method of contraception which has been developed in a variety of forms, including a nasal spray, is probably nearest of all the new methods of contraception to being made available.

Another option is to produce a vaccine which will immunize a woman against getting pregnant. Ideally this would make her immune to her husband's sperm or possibly to her own egg. An alternative to this would be to immunize a woman against proteins on the surface of a fertilized egg in the very earliest form of development before it has even attached itself to the womb. Other methods also depend on making the womb unreceptive to the fertilized egg. These methods are, in effect, abortifacient rather than contraceptive and may not be acceptable to some women, in spite of the fact that the intrauterine device is also thought to prevent implantation of the newly fertilized egg and this method is widely used.

The chances of an effective male Pill becoming available before the end of the century are remote. Scientists insist that it is much more difficult to devise a method of contraception to prevent formation of millions of sperm, compared with release of a single egg. And there is something in what they say, although many women argue that if it had been the men who had the children a safe and effective male Pill would have been found long before now! It is most unlikely that there will be any radically new forms of contraception available, even for women, before the end of this decade and even those at the most advanced stages of development are not without unwanted effects.

Anti-viral Drugs

As we have seen in an earlier chapter, viral diseases have long been the poor relations of the infectious-disease market. Bacteria may learn all too quickly how to overpower antibiotics developed to combat them but viruses have largely had a clear field with few if any drugs capable of getting at them.

Since viruses actually insert themselves inside the genetic material of the human cell any developments in anti-viral drugs must aim to prevent the viral particles from reproducing while at the same time avoiding any interference with the normal functions of the cell's own genes. Scientists have had some success at this, particularly with drugs to combat the herpes group of viruses which cause cold sores, eye and genital infections. In some of these the drug kills the virus while in others it boosts the body's immune cells to deal with the infection. But there are enormous gaps in the treatment of many viral conditions, from the common cold to hepatitis and, most recently, AIDS. Advances in the understanding of viral genes and how they reproduce is making it easier to develop new drugs but it will be many years before the lists of anti-viral drugs come anywhere near to the length of those for bacterial infections.

Vaccines

Ideally, scientists would like to eradicate the most severe infections altogether. Flushed with its success in eradicating smallpox in 1979, the World Health Organization looked to its other targets: tuberculosis, diphtheria, polio, malaria, typhoid and cholera. But the chances of success here are more remote, not least because of the sheer volume of people needing vaccination. While the emphasis is on producing safer vaccines for infections widely experienced in Britain, people in developing countries are a long way from having the same protection against their common infections.

Work is in progress on a safer whooping-cough vaccine and on a vaccine against herpes. But in Africa alone, one million children die from malaria each year and thousands more from bilharzia and sleeping sickness. Even a vaccine against leprosy is not yet available and many people still suffer needless debility and disfigurement from the infection because they cannot afford the drugs which are available.

Vaccine development has benefited enormously from the arrival of genetic engineering. In the past, vaccines came in two forms. Either they contained the killed whole organism or they contained part of the live bacterium or virus. Both methods had their drawbacks. The killed organisms might not be able to trigger a sufficient response from the body's immune system for it to be able to remember and recognize future attacks. But the live vaccine, in spite of frequently containing only part of the organism, ran the risk of causing nearly as bad an attack of the infection as the real thing.

The crucial part of the organism needed for the vaccine is the protein generally on the surface of the organism which is capable of triggering the protective response of the immune system. In the past, scientists were not able to collect these specific proteins and frequently landed themselves with other dangerous proteins which could attack the body. New techniques, an offshoot of the genetic engineering programmes under way around the world, have now enabled scientists to pinpoint much more accurately just the proteins they want. They are able to pull these off the virus or bacterium and put them in their vaccines. A number of vaccines are now well on the way to production thanks to these new techniques. And even the malaria parasite – whose complex lifecycle has always defeated previous vaccine development – is likely to fall to the modern techniques within the next few years.

Sadly, cost may prevent such vaccines getting to the very people who need them most. The malaria vaccine will be the culmination of twenty years of research by scientists all over the world and its cost will reflect the length of that research. While business people and travellers to exotic climes will be able to afford the vaccine, those who are exposed to the parasite every day of their lives in third-world countries will probably go on suffering from this potentially lethal infection because the cost of the vaccine will put it out of their reach.

Senility

The population over seventy-five years old in the United Kingdom is expected to have doubled by the year 2000. Most other western countries are also experiencing a massive surge in the number of their elderly people. What is to be done for all these people? Some will be crippled with arthritis, others with circulatory disease. But the biggest cause of chronic illness will be senility.

There is no cure for senility. Under the microscope the nerve cells in the brain take on the appearance of a tangled mass of fibres where once they were carefully networked. How to untangle them and just how important those tangles are in the degenerative process remains a mystery. The onset of the disease can be slow and insidious or sudden, often following a traumatic event such as the loss of a spouse or serious illness or injury. Unfortunately, the disease often gets worse when the patient goes into a long-stay ward of a hospital; someone who has managed to stay alert and independent for eighty years can suddenly degenerate into helplessness after even a few weeks in hospital.

Since it seemed that it was a deteriorating blood supply to the nerve cells in the brain which was at least contributing to the senility, drugs were developed in the Sixties and Seventies to dilate the blood vessels to the brain. But this seems to have little effect on the illness and attention has turned to the nerve degeneration rather than the blood supply in the search for a way of preventing or reversing senility.

Once again, drug advances can only follow a greater understanding of the disease process; and the nervous system, being one of the least understood areas of medicine, is ripe for basic research which can be made use of by drug companies in their search for drugs. A lot of attention has centred on deficiencies and over-production of the chemicals which transmit messages down the nerve cells. And the discovery that in contrast to previous scientific understanding some people can grow new nerve cells after they are damaged, or be taught to use previously unused cells, has given new fervour to the search for clues to senility.

When a breakthrough does come, as in time it must, drugs to prevent or treat senility will find a huge market – possibly larger than any so far. After all, no one wants to survive into their eighties and nineties unaware of what is going on around them and locked into a world unreached by family and friends.

CHAPTER 6

The Cost of Drugs

Do you know how much your drugs cost? The total drugs' bill in the United Kingdom makes up about 10 per cent of the cost of the NHS. The rest goes on staffing, buildings, hospital care, and general administration. But it still amounted to over £24 worth of drugs for every man, woman and child in the country in 1983 and is thought now to have reached the £30 mark. Too many prescriptions and the rising cost of drugs have combined to cause a massive increase in the drugs' bill over the last decade.

Drug prices vary enormously, from a few pence a day for a simple antibiotic to several hundred pounds for a single injection of one of the most powerful anti-cancer drugs. Of course, a lot depends on how long treatment is to go on for. A single dose of a common blood-pressure-lowering drug costs only 5p but as any one patient is likely to have to take it twice a day, seven days a week, 365 days of the year for the rest of his life, that cheap heart drug can work out far more expensive than something which costs more for each dose but is only used in short courses over four or five days.

In Britain, the most commonly prescribed group of drugs are the diuretics, used to lower blood pressure. They are relatively cheap, costing the taxpayer a mere £58 million a year. Less commonly prescribed are anti-inflammatory drugs for arthritis. But these are much more expensive and, at £124 million a year, they are more than double the cost of most other commonly used drugs.

Overseas, doctors appear to have different priorities. While we concentrate on our joints and blood pressure, the Italians and French are much more concerned about the condition of their digestive systems and spend far more than we do on drugs to combat abdominal conditions. Overall, we spend less on our health as a proportion of the gross national product (GNP) than virtually any other country in the world. The United States, West Germany, France, the Scandinavian countries, Australia and Japan all spend a greater proportion of GNP on health care than we do in Britain.

Even so, the cost of drugs has escalated to such a degree in recent years that the government has taken steps to reduce the total bill. The bill for drugs prescribed on the NHS rose from £209 million in 1970 to £1118 million in 1980 and a massive £1600 million by 1983. At that rate of increase, the bill will have topped the £2 billion mark in the next year or so. To offset the drugs' bill the government currently collects prescription charges from just under half the population. The charge for a prescription has increased from 45p per item in 1979 to £2 in 1985. But only one in four prescriptions are made out to people eligible for prescription charges; those who do not pay include the elderly and many of the chronically sick who tend to need more drugs than average.

It is not the number of prescriptions which has increased dramatically in the last fifteen years, however; it is the cost of the ingredients in each prescription. In 1970 there were 295 million prescriptions handed out to patients in the United Kingdom and the average cost of each item on those prescriptions was just 54p. By 1982 the number of prescriptions had increased to 370 million but the average cost of each ingredient had risen nearly sevenfold to £3.14.

Drugs were not the only goods to have increased so dramatically in price during that period. But, as cuts are being made elsewhere in the health service, it is obvious that savings also need to be made in the drugs' bill. The government has already taken steps to curtail drug-industry profits but what can doctors and consumers do to try and help reduce the drugs bill? After all, it is we who pay, whether directly through our prescription charges, or indirectly through our taxes.

How Are Drugs Priced?

Like most commodities, drugs are priced according to what the consumer will pay, the consumer in this case being the NHS. The price of a new drug will depend to some extent on the prices of rival drugs already on the market. Just as the manufacturers of a new form of bleach will not market it at a price twice that of similar products, so it is with new drugs. If the company feels it has strong grounds for promoting its product as far superior to other drugs for the same disease it might introduce it at a higher price and then go all out to convince doctors of its superior merits. And if it has got a real breakthrough on its hands then the sky is the limit. With no competing products the company can charge the most it feels it can get away with.

Setting a high price early on is not always in a company's interests however. If its balance sheets at the end of the year record massive profits out of all proportion to the company's turnover the government may require it to pay some money back.

Each year all companies which sell more than £1.5 million worth of drugs to the DHSS have to submit details of their turnover, profits and losses to a body within the DHSS which decides on the increase in prices which each company can charge in the following year. Every company has a different amount of allowable profit although the DHSS is currently aiming to limit this to 16 per cent of turnover. As the costs of raw materials, running costs and salaries rise, the drug companies are allowed to increase their prices to maintain the agreed profit level. This does not mean that all their drugs rise by the same amount; companies keep watch on what rival firms are doing and in some years they may limit their price increases to one range of products and, in another, concentrate on an entirely different range.

The amount of allowable profit is not based solely on the rising costs of running a drug company. Firms score 'brownie points' according to their track record of the previous year. If, for example, they have built a new factory or increased their work-force or developed a really innovative drug they are allowed a higher profit margin than a company which has not invested in British skills and work-force. So, although the target profit allowable for companies on the whole may be set at 16 per cent, companies which have been particularly 'good' can have their profit allowance more than doubled. But if a company goes way beyond its allowable profit margin it will have to pay the extra profits back and will not be allowed to increase its prices the following year.

All industries whose major customer is a government department have profit limits laid down according to the risk in the industry. These limits are not legally binding. The pharmaceutical industry is considered to be a relatively high-risk industry since it undertakes the research and development of new drugs without any guarantees of success or return on investment. Other industries which will always have a guaranteed market for their products and do not have to risk large amounts of money in research and development are allowed smaller profit margins.

The price-regulation scheme currently in force in Britain was drawn up in 1978 jointly by the Department of Health and the pharmaceutical industry. It remains voluntary but all companies with more than the minimum allowable turnover use it. The aim is to strike a careful balance between allowing sufficient profits to drug companies to encourage them to remain based in Britain, bringing with them investment and employment, and allowing too much profit, which would lead to the NHS finding itself paying ever-increasing bills for the drugs consumed in hospitals and prescribed by general practitioners.

The body which controls the pricing scheme, based as it is within the DHSS, has an unenviable task. It has been argued that the job should not be carried out at the DHSS since it involves conflicting interests. One alternative would be for the Department of Trade to bargain on behalf of the industry in order to improve profits for companies while the DHSS should consider only its own interest, namely to keep drugs cheap for the NHS. In this way the Departments of Trade and Health would negotiate the deal for the industry between them, instead of the DHSS in effect having to negotiate on its own and the industry's behalf as at present.

Some countries have legally binding price limits for their drugs. In France for example the government keeps prices down and in Belgium, too, prices are lower than in the United Kingdom. In some cases, the price differentials are so big that it is cheaper for drug distributors to re-import British-made drugs from European countries. Even when the transportation and administrative costs are added on, the drugs are cheaper when bought in Europe than if they were bought here.

In recent years, the profit margins of the drug industry in Britain have come under close scrutiny from the powerful House of Commons Committee of Public Accounts. This is an all-party committee which, from time to time, checks up where money allocated by Parliament for public expenditure actually gets spent. Twice it has looked at the drug industry's profits and twice it has recommended decreases in the amounts allowed. The government, while not implementing the full decreases recommended, has reduced profit limits and disallowed price rises.

Restricted Lists

At the end of 1984, the government introduced a plan which it hoped would cut around £100 million off the drugs bill. The idea was to reduce the number of products available on the NHS in eight categories of drug. These were antacids for indigestion, laxatives for constipation, inhalations and antitussives for coughs and colds, analgesics for mild to moderate pain, vitamins, tonics and benzodiazepine sleeping pills and tranquillizers. Rarely has there been such a howl of protest from the drug industry and the medical profession in the forty-year history of the NHS.

Both groups claimed that the scheme would lead to a two-tier system of health care for rich and poor. Those who could afford to pay would be able to continue getting their favourite medicines while those without the money would have to make do with what the NHS was prepared to offer. The drug industry mounted a massive advertising campaign which elicited some 100,000 letters of support from worried patients. The medical profession refused to negotiate over the contents of the blacklist; the DHSS had made its bed, now it could lie in it, was the thinking. By introducing its plan without warning and allowing only two months for consultation, health ministers could have expected a stormy ride. But even they must have been surprised at the vehemence of the response from the drug industry and the medical profession.

It was not that the idea of restricting the number of drugs available was new. Hospitals all over the country had been implementing their own voluntary lists for several years. These had been drawn up after lengthy discussions between consultants and pharmacologists and doctors were generally free to override the list if they felt sufficiently strongly that their patient needed a specific drug not on the list; experience showed that they rarely did.

In some areas the list spread from the local hospital to general practice. It made sense that patients on certain drugs when they left hospital should continue on them when they returned to the care of their GP. And many hard-pressed family doctors were glad of guidance as to the most cost-effective drugs from their hospital colleagues, in view of the vast amount of promotional literature with which they were faced each day.

As a compromise with the DHSS, the British Medical Association (BMA) proposed that if the official blacklist plan were withdrawn they would organize local committees of doctors to draw up lists of drugs for GPs which could be used on a voluntary basis similar to what was already happening in some parts of the country. But this was not enough for the DHSS; the drugs' bill was rocketing, to over £1600 million annually, and it wanted immediate action.

In view of the BMA's refusal to negotiate, an advisory committee was set up to discuss necessary deductions from the blacklist to arrive at a more generally acceptable list when it was implemented on April 1 1985. In the event, the number of drugs on the list of allowed medicines in the eight categories was more than trebled, from thirty to one hundred different products and the government conceded that its expected savings from the scheme would fall from £100 million to £75 million. Many observers argued that the savings would be considerably less than that.

With many of their favourite drugs back on the so-called 'white list' of products which could now be prescribed on the NHS, it seemed as though the campaign by the doctors and drug industry had paid off. But although health ministers have promised that no other groups of drugs will get the blacklist treatment for the time being there is little doubt that they have their collective eye on a number of other drugs whose restriction could make the current £75 million saving seem like a drop in the ocean.

A reduction in the number of blood pressure and anti-inflammatory drugs, contraceptive pills and antibiotics could really send the drugs' bill tumbling. But is the current blacklist really causing the decline in patient care forecast by the medical profession and the drug industry? Are we really suffering from the reduction in numbers of drugs available to treat our indigestion, constipation, coughs and colds, anxiety and insomnia? Or was it all a storm in a teacup deliberately blown up by a medical profession determined to protect its freedom to prescribe what it likes and a drug industry set on preserving its profits?

How the Blacklist of Drugs has Affected Patients

One thing is certain: in the weeks and months after the introduction of the limited list there was no massive upsurge in the number of private prescriptions. Few patients, deprived of their regular drugs but offered an NHS alternative for which they would not have to pay, felt the urge to dig into their pockets and fork out for a private prescription of their old medicine. Neither doctors nor pharmacists reported any of the chaos and confusion amongst patients forecast in some quarters for the start of the scheme. Was it just that the long-suffering patient had got used to the privations of Tory rule or were the alternative drugs now available perfectly acceptable to both doctor and patient?

There is no doubt that the original list had left off some important drugs. It omitted certain important antacids for people who regurgitate stomach acid; it left patients with chronic constipation with only two somewhat outdated laxatives, not designed to cope with the various intestinal abnormalities which can cause constipation; one of the most famous – and controversial – pain-killers, Distalgesic, was not to be available in any form and some of the latest tranquillizers and sleeping pills, with fewest side-effects, were blacklisted while older benzodiazepines with more side-effects remained. A handful of important vitamin combinations were missing but no one could seriously mourn the passing of dozens of other vitamins, tonics and cough and cold remedies more suited to the over-the-counter trade than the prescription pad.

By the time the new list was published, virtually all of the drugs which were acknowledged to have a real medical place, yet which had been blacklisted, were restored to the categories of prescribable drugs on the NHS. In a handful of cases, where patients had been established with difficulty on an effective drug which turned out to be blacklisted, there was real cause for such patients to be able to continue with their banned medications. People do respond differently to drugs and if they have tried everything else there seems to be good reason to allow them to continue on the only thing that works.

Will a Restricted List Really Lower Prices?

Of all the options open to it, the government chose a restricted list to cut drug costs because it thought this would achieve the biggest saving. But it has already lost £25 million in savings, simply by expanding the 'white list'.

Before making their decision, health ministers had looked carefully at list systems enforced abroad, and at the savings already achieved in British hospitals. A number of countries have systems whereby patients are reimbursed different proportions of the costs of their drugs according to the importance of the medicine. For example, in Belgium patients pay nothing for life-saving drugs, 25 per cent for important drugs, 50 per cent of the cost of less-than-useful products and the full amount for medicines considered to be of no therapeutic value. Similarly, in France they pay 60 per cent of the cost of drugs for mild conditions, 30 per cent for homeopathic medicines and essential drugs for twenty-four listed conditions are free.

West Germany has one of the newest list systems for reimbursement of drugs and it bears distinct similarities to our own. Included on a blacklist containing non-reimbursable drugs are tonics, laxatives, cough and cold remedies, minor pain-killers, vitamins, antacids, rubs and inhalations, travel-sickness and slimming preparations. The scheme was met with widespread criticism when it was introduced in 1983 and it is claimed that projected savings have simply not materialized.

Here at home, variable savings have been made at different hospitals with the introduction of lists of prescribable drugs. One of the first lists was introduced at Ninewells hospital, in Dundee. It contained only 193 drugs and in the first year caused a saving of 7.5 per cent in the drugs bill. In Nottingham, £10,000, has been lopped off the drugs bill at the university hospital as a result of more cost-effective prescribing. In some cases the drugs bill has not fallen, but its rate of increase has been halted so that costs have remained stable. It seems inevitable that prices will go up year by year; the important thing is to halt the exponential increases of recent years and put the trend back towards the much steadier increases of ten to fifteen years ago.

An interesting experiment at a London health centre has shown that drugs costs can be reduced in general practice too. The private Harrow Health Care Centre which was started in 1982 charges patients just over £100 a year for all medical care and drugs they may require. Patients pay an annual subscription. The Centre operates a list of 600 drugs and doctors use generic rather than brand-named drugs for between 50 and 60 per cent of their prescriptions. The director of the Centre explains that only top-quality British-made generics are used and foreign-made drugs of dubious origin studiously avoided. On top of these cost-cutting exercises doctors at the practice only prescribe the number of tablets which their patients need, rather than standard quantities of thirty, fifty or more tablets. Frequently patients go away with only five or six tablets since this is all that doctors believe they need. It has been calculated that these measures together have saved the health centre between £4 and £5 per patient per year. It may not sound a great deal but it has been estimated that a similar saving nationwide would add up to nearly £300 million.

Immediate savings on the drugs bill was not the only intention behind the introduction of the limited list. By drawing up black and white lists of drugs the government has not closed the door for ever on companies whose products are disallowed. It has set up a committee to assess whether new drugs are sufficiently cost-effective to merit inclusion on the 'white list' and to review changing prices of established drugs to see whether they are sufficiently cheap to get on the NHS list.

Companies whose drugs were placed on the blacklist have already taken steps to price them more competitively. In many cases branded drugs are now the same price as the cheap generic alternatives prescribable on the NHS and in some instances companies have actually dropped the trade names of their products and are marketing them alongside the generics. The pharmacist, who simply buys the cheapest available version of a drug for the NHS list, is now finding that previously expensive trade-named products are the cheapest variety around. This dramatic fall in prices of some household name drugs such as Mogadon, Dalmane and Tranxene begs the question: if companies can afford to set such low prices now why did they not do it before. Has the NHS been ripped off?

Trade Names Versus Generics

In deciding to go for a restricted-list system, the government tossed aside an alternative solution to the escalating drugs bill favoured by the British Medical Association – generic prescribing. Health ministers felt that even generic prescribing right across all categories of drug would not yield a sufficient saving. And, although it favoured the principle of generic prescribing, the BMA wanted it left to individual doctors to decide when they were prepared for a generic drug to be dispensed and they were not prepared for it to be left to the pharmacist to take responsibility for substituting a generic version automatically.

What is a generic drug? Every drug that comes on to the market has three names – the chemical name (generally unpronounceable and referring to the chemical structure of the compound), the generic name (marginally more pronounceable and the drug's 'common' name) and its trade name (the name bestowed by the manufacturer on its latest brainchild). Thus, the chemical name for the common tranquillizer Valium is 7-chloro-1,3-dihydro-1-methyl-5-phenyl-2H-1,4-benzodiazepin-2-ONE. Its generic name is diazepam and Valium is its trade name.

Trade-named or branded drugs are almost invariably more

expensive than generic drugs, sometimes by a few pence, often by several pounds. The difference is frequently likened to famous name and own brand consumer goods such as baked beans. Heinz beans are more expensive than those made by chain-store supermarkets, for example.

When it comes to consumer goods, the reason for the price difference is often only too obvious. Foods may not taste so good, clothes may be less stylish. But all drugs have to meet the same standards of safety and quality, whether they are marketed generically or by their trade name. So when we buy Valium rather than diazepam or Inderal instead of propranolol what are we paying the extra for? Some of the extra cost reflects the investment in researching and developing the branded drug which got it to the market in the first place. Companies which sell generic drugs do not research and develop their own products but market other people's drugs once the patent runs out.

As soon as a drug company thinks it has found a winning drug, it obtains a patent for the chemical to prevent other companies from working on it and getting it on to the market first. This is standard practice in any industry. Computer manufacturers patent their latest microchip, chocolate manufacturers their latest syrup, even biologists patent the cells they are working on. Drug companies have to time their patent application very carefully because once it is in black and white the clock starts ticking and they have twenty years in which to make their profit. Once the patent runs out other companies are free to market their own version of the same chemical and compete for the market by dropping the price of the drug.

Twenty years sounds long enough to make a splendid return on the cost of researching and developing the product. And so it is for discoveries in some industries. But when you remember that it can take up to ten years to get a drug through all its safety tests and on to the market this leaves only ten years to rake in the profits. Indeed, the drug industry argues that, on latest estimates, companies are left with less than nine years to market their drugs free from competition, such is the time taken up by safety testing and delays in licensing. So it is crucial for the drug company to time its patent just right. Too early and it will not leave long enough for the company to recoup its investment; too late, and a rival company will get in first and patent the chemical for itself.

In the earliest days, drugs generally took their names from their manufacturers. Thus, we had such quaint drugs as Clarke's blood mixture, De Witt's analgesic pills, Dr Williams' pink pills and Jenners' suspension. Once the major drug companies grew to their present size and were producing hundreds of drugs apiece they had to be rather more imaginative. And they chose names for their drugs which tried to put across the message of the drug. Thus, Fortral – a pain-killer – gives a feel of power and strength; Librium – a sleeping pill – puts across a tranquil image, free of troubles and the name Marvelon – a contraceptive pill – speaks for itself. More recently companies have spent more time searching their computers for names that have not already been used than dreaming up really novel names. A company must also bear in mind foreign sensitivities if a drug is to be sold worldwide.

Once the patent on a drug runs out, any drug company can market it, either giving it a new trade name or marketing it under its generic name. Thus the tranquillizer diazepam was marketed by its discoverer, Roche, as Valium, as Alupram by a company called Steinhard, Atensine by Berk, Diazemuls by KabiVitrum, Evacalm by Unimed, Solis by Galen, Stesolid by CP Pharm, Tensium by a firm called DDSA and as Valrelease, also by Roche. One drug, nine names. Today it is only available on the NHS in its generic version, diazepam.

Certain companies in Britain specialize in making generic drugs, others are subsidiaries of large companies which also do their own research and development. Glaxo is one of these. It both researches new drugs as Glaxo and manufactures generics through one of its subsidiaries.

When drug companies manufacturing trade-named drugs are criticized for charging such high prices for their drugs they argue that they must charge more in order to recoup their investment so that they can put money into future research. Generic companies, they say, are riding on the backs of the big research companies, letting them do all the hard work and waiting for patents to run out on major drugs. They are not prepared to put their own money up front in the risky and expensive business of research and development.

But the fact remains that if you are faced with two identical products and one is priced £5, £10, £15 more than the other you are not going to choose the more expensive brand just because its manufacturer produced the drug first. So it is with the NHS; with a drugs' bill in excess of £1.5 billion per year, it was hardly surprising that successive health ministers examined the prospect of introducing more widespread mandatory generic prescribing.

Many of the drugs on the limited list are cheaper generic versions of the original trade-named products. And where generic versions are not available and branded products are prescribable, manufacturers have been given due warning that, as soon as a generic version is available, the branded version will be blacklisted unless the manufacturer can offer it at a competitive price.

Are We Getting the Best Drugs?

More widespread generic prescribing does not mean that we are getting sub-standard drugs. As already mentioned, British generic manufacturers have to meet the same high safety standards as manufacturers of branded drugs. The same is not always true of drugs imported from abroad. Isolated cases have occurred of imported drugs not meeting British standards and the onus is on importers and pharmacists to ensure that they know exactly where their drugs have come from and that standards are met.

The way in which a drug is released from its formulation – be it tablet, capsule, linctus or cream – does vary between formulations produced by different manufacturers. And in a handful of cases where it is crucial that patients receive their drugs in exactly the same format it is important that they continue to receive the same product from the same manufacturer. But this is indeed rare and the drugs concerned are well known.

Even before the government started to restrict the number of drugs available on the NHS, some doctors had introduced prescribing policies into their own practices, frequently based on the more widespread use of generic drugs. A detailed study in 1980 which involved over fifty doctors showed that GPs can reduce the cost of their prescribing when potential savings are pointed out to them. All the prescriptions which a doctor writes out find their way to a central collecting house in Newcastle after they are dispensed by the pharmacist. There, the cost of each drug on each prescription is worked out so that pharmacists can be reimbursed for the cost of the drugs they have dispensed. At the same time, records are kept of each doctor's prescribing costs. Once a year each GP is sent a print-out comparing the cost of his prescriptions with the average for his area. But he will only get a detailed breakdown of his prescribing in each category of drug if the cost of his prescriptions is excessively high. If his costs are 50 per cent more than his local colleagues he is taken to task and shown the error of his ways. As he receives a detailed record of the cost of the drugs he has prescribed, he can see where he is overprescribing.

It is hoped that once the Newcastle system is fully computerized, these detailed analyses will be sent out not just to erring doctors but to all GPs in the country. It was these detailed charts which were used in the 1980 study to see if doctors who were told more about exactly what they had prescribed could be persuaded to reduce the cost of their prescriptions.

The doctors in the study were divided into three groups. In the first group were GPs whose prescribing habits were thought to be relatively well trained already, because they were in close contact with hospital colleagues specializing in cost-effective prescribing. In the second group were doctors chosen at random who were neither big prescribers nor particularly cost-conscious. The third group of doctors was a 'control' group, who were not advised about reducing their drugs and were included so that any improvements in the other groups could be compared with their own unchanged prescribing habits.

The doctors in the study were given regular breakdowns of the type of drug they prescribed and what it cost. They attended seminars and were given information-packs about their own prescribing and that of their practice as a whole. At the meetings, the doctors were told about the generic equivalents of the drugs they had prescribed, and discussed the relative costs and effectiveness of these drugs as well as those situations where drugs might be avoided.

The study lasted a total of eighteen months and at the end of that time the doctors' prescribing habits were compared with those at the beginning of the study. The number of items prescribed per

1000 patients fell by 8.5 per cent in the randomly collected doctors and by over 15 per cent in those who were assumed to be more cost-effective prescribers in the first place. But there was a reduction of only 3 per cent in the control group. When the costs were compared, they were found to have gone up in all the groups, which might seem surprising at first glance but was, of course, inevitable as prices rose generally over the eighteen months. What was reassuring was the fact that the increase in cost was much lower in both groups who had attended seminars and been given information about their prescribing than in the control doctors. The study showed first that there are significant savings to be made in the drugs prescribed by GPs, and it also showed that doctors are prepared to prescribe fewer and cheaper drugs when they are given detailed figures about their prescribing.

The doctors who ran the study decided to check whether the GPs continued their better prescribing once the study had ended. Unfortunately, three years on, they had reverted to their previous, more expensive, habits. And it seems that, like anyone else, doctors need feedback about how they are doing. Show them the figures and they can see where there is room for improvement, which drugs can be reduced and where cheaper alternatives will do the job just as well. But if they cannot see what they are prescribing and only get an annual report comparing their overall performance to that of other local doctors they find it much harder to stay on the straight and narrow.

In general, doctors jealously guard their right to prescribe what they think suitable, invoking their right to clinical freedom. Drugs are licensed for the treatment of specific diseases, but doctors may prescribe them for whatever illness they see fit, provided they are prepared to take responsibility for their actions. Thus if they wanted to, they could prescribe a heart drug for a chest infection or a tranquillizer for diabetes. Naturally, they would not have a legal leg to stand on if the patient died as a result of a misguided prescription. (The drug company would not be held responsible because it only promoted the drug for conditions where it had a licence.) This may seem a strange right, but one of the reasons for clinical freedom in prescribing is to enable doctors to use their skill and experience to try a drug for a different non-licensed disease, if they genuinely think it might do some good.

All kinds of new uses for old drugs have been discovered by doctors trying them out. Even dangerous drugs may have their uses in very special circumstances. For example, only a few years ago, and long after it was officially withdrawn from the market, doctors discovered that thalidomide was a very useful drug for the treatment of a debilitating disease which has very serious mouth ulcers as one of its symptoms. Provided there is no risk of the patients getting pregnant there is no reason why even this drug cannot be used to treat a condition where no other effective treatment is available.

But some are now asking whether this clinical freedom has outlived its usefulness. The government has already put some curb on this tradition by introducing its restricted list, and doctors abiding by local lists of their own have also abdicated some of that freedom. Clinical freedom came in with the introduction of the NHS in 1948 but almost forty years on we must look again at whether we can still afford such a luxury.

It is not simply a question of cutting costs, it is also a matter of moving with the times. The term used is cost-effective prescribing and the 'effective' part is just as important. Do we want to be fobbed off with medicines we do not need or which are not effective? Or would we prefer that savings be made on unnecessary medicines so that the money could be spent on drugs to treat life-threatening or chronic, serious illness?

'We had a woman in recently with prescriptions for drugs for arthritis. In two weeks she came in with four or five different prescriptions. We discovered that she was going to a different doctor in the same practice and none of them knew what had already been prescribed. She would try the drug for a day or two, decide it didn't work and go back to the doctor for something different. By the time we told the doctors what was happening they had prescribed over £160 worth of drugs.'

A pharmacist

How Can We Help to Lower the Drugs Bill?

Keeping the drugs bill down is not the responsibility of just the medical profession and the drug industry. We too can and should play our part in reducing costs – not least because it is we who will pick up the bill at the end of the day, through our taxes.

We have to rely on our doctors to advise on what drugs we should take but they frequently take their cue from us. Some patients make it clear from the outset that they will not be satisfied to leave the surgery without a prescription while others try to avoid drugs unless they are really necessary. A few refuse all drugs – and that is their decision.

Any figure for the number of unnecessary prescriptions handed out each year has to be an estimate. But some clue may come from doctors' prescribing habits. On average, doctors give prescriptions to two out of three patients who come and see them; however, some doctors have reduced this to one in two patients – a fall of 16 per cent, equivalent to 39 million prescriptions if it were applied nationwide. Patients whose doctors have reduced their prescribing do not seem to have suffered without those extra prescriptions. So why do more doctors not reduce the number of drugs they hand out?

There is no doubt that the prescription-pad is the easy option. It takes far less time to write a prescription than to explain why a drug is not needed. The general assumption that there is a pill for every ill is so deep-rooted that it will take a long time to persuade people that they do not need a drug for every ache and pain, cough and cold.

In the height of summer over 100,000 people consult their doctor each week with a sore throat, and in the winter that figure more than doubles. What are they all doing there? What miracle cure are they looking for? Coughs, colds and sore throats are thought to be responsible for more unnecessary prescriptions than any other form of illness. But the truth of the matter remains that there is no cure for any of these problems and drugs can only relieve symptoms. These are just as well bought from the chemist and frequently cost less than the price of a prescription. The government blacklist has put a tough restriction on just which of these remedies are available on the NHS.

Many people, though, want more than just sympathy and cough-mixture for their cold; they also want, and frequently get, an antibiotic. In 1982, some forty-six million prescriptions were issued for antibiotics putting them third only to drugs used to treat diseases of the nervous system and circulatory disorders. The image of the antibiotic as the cure-all for every infection lives on, in spite of the fact that there are armies of organisms which are totally impervious to such drugs, including the viruses which cause colds and the vast majority of sore throats.

Antibiotics are used to treat bacterial infections and bacteria resemble viruses about as much as a cauliflower resembles a tadpole. Most gastric and urinary infections are caused by bacteria, as are whooping cough, typhoid, tetanus, meningitis and gonorrhoea. Colds, flu, measles, mumps, chicken-pox and shingles are all caused by viruses and do not respond to antibiotics.

In general, viral infections are more difficult to treat than bacterial infections and far fewer drugs are available. While bacteria attack cells from the outside, viruses are able to get into the very heart of the cell and reproduce themselves alongside the cell's own genetic material. Fortunately, the cells do get wise to this intrusion and expel the foreign material and the common viral infections, like those caused by bacteria, are frequently self-limiting; in a few days the symptoms disappear and the patient feels better.

Drugs are needed for the more severe infections and antibiotics and anti-viral drugs can be lifesavers, so long as they are each used to treat the infections for which they were designed.

For years, doctors have prescribed antibiotics for throat infections, few of which needed them. The usual justification for this is that they wish to treat any secondary infection which may have arisen. But what they are really doing is keeping the customer satisfied; the patient comes in for an antibiotic and that is what he gets. Secondary infections in the throat caused by bacteria are rare and it is impossible to decide whether a sore throat is caused by a viral or a bacterial infection just by looking at it. Throat swabs sent to the laboratory would give the answer but it is simply not cost-effective to check the cause of every sore throat – which will probably clear up in a few days anyway.

The chances of a secondary bacterial infection which would respond to antibiotic treatment increase if the sore throat persists for more than seven days. And the likelihood of a bacterial cause for the infection increases if the patient has a high fever. But a basic rule of thumb is that if you can get to the surgery with your throat it is probably a viral, not a bacterial, infection, just as if you can get to work you have got a cold, not flu.

Does it really matter that we are being prescribed antibiotics for viral infections? Is it not better to be safe than sorry?

It is not just a question of cost. Unnecessary use of antibiotics increases the risk of bacteria becoming resistant to these drugs. So when they are given to patients with serious bacterial infections who really need them, they simply do not work. The bacteria recognize the antibiotic and overpower it. Each time we take an antibiotic for a mild sore throat we are pushing up the chances of it not working when we need it most.

Dozens of antibiotics have been developed since the first penicillins in the 1930s. Some are designed to work against a wide range of bacteria, others have a much narrower range of activity and are effective against only a handful of organisms. It is tempting for doctors to prescribe the newer, and generally more expensive, broad-spectrum antibiotics which are designed to work against a number of different bacteria. But experts agree that in the majority of cases the older, cheaper, narrow-spectrum drugs should be used because they are less likely to cause resistance to develop.

The cost of antibiotics and the risk of serious infections are not the only reasons for not pressing your doctor for drugs for more minor and generally self-limiting infections. There is also the time factor. We have already seen how difficult it is for many patients to discuss their problems in the space of the average five-minute consultation. Anxiety, depression and other emotional problems are not easily solved in such a short time. But doctors could spend more time with such patients if those with minor throat infections went to the chemist for drugs to relieve their symptoms instead of going to their doctor for antibiotics.

The onus is not solely on the patient. Doctors frequently do not take the time to explain why drugs are not needed, and patients go away feeling that their problem has not been taken seriously. This is not true just of coughs and colds. Numerous aches and pains have no obvious basis, and while they cause the sufferer considerable discomfort, they frequently disappear within a week or so of their own accord; aspirin or paracetamol provide a more suitable treatment than the expensive anti-inflammatory drugs that are frequently prescribed and that should be reserved for chronic arthritic-type pain.

A radical change in attitude on the part of both doctors and patients is vital if a much-needed reduction in the number of drugs being prescribed is to be achieved. Doctors must take time to explain to their patients why they do not need drugs and patients must be prepared to listen. Patients deserve to feel re-assured that their problem has been taken seriously, and that they can come back if it persists and they remain convinced that treatment is needed.

All too often, the patient's ability to understand what is wrong is underestimated by both doctor and patient alike. Or the doctor falls back on medical jargon which is totally incomprehensible to anyone who is not medically qualified – and quite a few who are. Sometimes she does this because she does not know what is wrong with her patient and does not like to admit it; and at other times she uses jargon because she cannot be bothered to simplify things for her patient.

But if there is to be any chance of reducing the number and cost of drugs used in the NHS, doctor and patient must work together to achieve a more rational use of drugs. The responsibility lies with neither party alone and each will be faced with the bill.

Will Cost-cutting Ruin the Drug Industry?

British drug exports rose by 14 per cent in 1984 to an all-time high of £1.2 billion. Imports also rose, by 15 per cent to £542 million, leaving a trade surplus of £680 million. This too was an increase on the previous year. Only America and Switzerland have more attractive figures to show their investors.

Britain has six major drug companies doing research and development for new products. It also has a number of smaller companies making generics or specializing in household products, with just a few drugs to keep their hand in. On top of these, a number of major European and American companies do research in this country. The result is that around 72,000 people work for drug firms in the United Kingdom.

The drug industry in Britain has quite a reputation for crying wolf. So often have they predicted the demise of their industry over the last ten years, that they have found it hard to find sympathy in their latest skirmish with the government over the restricted list. In spite of regular industry surveys into public attitudes, showing that we have great confidence in our drug producers, there can be few industries with a poorer image. Even arms dealers have an easier time, perhaps because they keep a lower profile. Small wonder that the drug industry is given to paranoia.

But is the industry headed for a slump in spite of its apparently healthy trade figures? Will the limited list, greater generic prescribing and reduced profits really put the final nails in the British drug industry's coffin and send American and European firms in search of new research bases where the economic climate is more favourable?

If there was a simple yes or no answer, there would be no controversy. If the industry were about to go under, the government would hardly be taking measures to finish off an important contributor to its balance of payments. Yet the drug industry can point at other countries that have lost their pharmaceutical firms because of stringent measures to reduce their profitability.

Australia and Canada are two such countries. The Australian government has imposed strict price controls on the drugs paid for under the equivalent of its NHS. The result has been that foreign drug companies have pulled out and no longer research or produce drugs locally. Drugs are imported and, having reduced their local overheads, the firms can provide drugs at the prices required by the government.

Canada has a generic-prescribing policy and pharmacists are encouraged to substitute generic drugs wherever appropriate. In addition, there is less patent protection of new drugs than occurs in Britain. Again, pharmaceutical firms have pulled out and very little research is done in Canada. Both Canada and Australia are thus importers rather than exporters of drugs and they have a negative trade balance.

In recent years, price controls have also been placed on drugs sold in some European countries, such as France and Belgium, and most French firms have now been nationalized. But it is too early to say what effect this will have on the industry in these countries. The Labour party has already said that any future government it controls will nationalize at least a part of the British drug industry. So, if drug firms feel hard done by under a Tory government, they may feel considerably more uneasy about a Labour government.

But can the situation in Britain be compared with that in Canada, Australia, France or Belgium? Britain has one of the highest reputations for the innovative skills of its researchers and the standards of care given by its doctors. It has a long tradition of coming up with the so-called breakthrough drugs. At present it comes second only to the United States in the number of products it has in the international top hundred best-selling drugs.

You can persuade a few hot-shot scientists to leave Britain and continue their research where conditions are more economically favourable, but you cannot uproot whole hospitals where doctors perform clinical trials of new drugs to the highest standards. And even if you could withdraw your research and development facilities, where are you going to put them? Britain is not the only country which has taken steps to reduce its drugs bill and limit industry profits. Most European countries, where many of the leading drug companies such as Hoechst, Bayer and Rocher are based, are also taking steps to curb drug prices and limit prescribing.

Some companies have already cancelled investment plans in the United Kingdom or have threatened to withdraw personnel and sell off factories and laboratories. But while there is so much uncertainty about the savings which will be made from the limited list and further measures with which the government plans directly to curb drug industry profitability, most firms are marking time. The fact that many firms are reducing their prices to compete with generic alternatives, in spite of the fact that this could have repercussions on prices in Europe and America, suggests that they are preparing to weather the storm. Or perhaps it was not the cyclone they had led us to believe.

CHAPTER 7

Drugs: Can We Do without Them?

At least one in five people will have taken a tranquillizer at some time in their lives. Some may have taken it just once, others for more than twenty years; they may still be taking it or they may be trying to stop. Rarely has the need to reduce the number of drugs we take been more obvious than during the epidemic of tranquillizer and sleeping-pill misuse of the Sixties and Seventies, which has still not been cured.

There is no typical tranquillizer taker. The image of the bored housewife moving from sherry to pill-bottle is false. True, more women than men take tranquillizers, but they seem just as likely to go out to work as to stay at home. A lot of confusion surrounds the difference between a tranquillizer and a sleeping pill. This is because they both come from the same family of drugs, called benzodiazepines. These are the most widely used group of drugs to treat anxiety and insomnia. Until the first benzodiazepine came on to the market in 1960, doctors prescribed barbiturates to calm people and help them sleep. These were soon recognized as addictive and people frequently used them to commit suicide. So there was a collective sigh of relief from the medical profession when the benzodiazepines were discovered. They were effective, remarkably free from side-effects and difficult to use for suicide, and they appeared not to be addictive.

The result was that in their peak years – the mid-Seventies – over forty million prescriptions were written each year in the United Kingdom for this group of drugs. An arbitrary distinction was drawn between benzodiazepines prescribed for anxiety and those used for insomnia. In fact, all the drugs are very similar; doses are higher at night since more of the drug is needed to induce sleep than merely to relieve anxiety. Some drugs have longer-lasting effects than others and these are more suited to the sixteen-hour day of the tranquillizer than the eight-hour night of the sleeping pill. The shorter-acting drugs are better as sleeping pills because they are less likely to make people wake up feeling hung over and sleepy during the day.

Thus, diazepam is a longer-acting drug and best suited to the treatment of anxiety and temazepam is shorter-acting and more geared to insomnia. But nitrazepam, which is long-acting, is widely used as a sleeping pill when its properties make it more suited to treating anxiety. Some years ago an advisory committee to the DHSS drew attention to such anomalies and recommended that drug companies think more carefully about the conditions for which they promote their benzodiazepines. But this has had little effect.

What Is Anxiety?

Everyone gets anxious from time to time; it is a natural response to stress. We all use it to our own advantage to enable us to do things we would think impossible in the cold light of day. There are plenty of actors and actresses, politicians and public speakers who say that they cannot perform unless they can feel the adrenalin pumping through their veins.

Anxiety can also be a warning sign to slow down. Stress is all very well in small doses but keep up the pressure for too long and you could be in for a shock – stomach ulcers, emotional upset, heart attack. We all have different things which make us anxious. A particular job which makes one person very anxious will seem like a piece of cake to someone else. But that same person who handles an important meeting with such ease may be climbing up the wall before an informal dinner party.

Common symptoms of anxiety include racing heartbeat, dizziness, breathing problems, a choking sensation, feelings of weakness in the arms and legs, nervous shaking, sweating, aches and pains and insomnia. People may appear tense and nervy, bad-tempered towards their friends and enemies alike and find it hard to concentrate.

What is normal anxiety for one person may be quite unacceptable to another. Which is why it can be very difficult to gauge whether someone is simply 'going through a bad patch' or is really disturbed. Some people seem to be naturally over-anxious and live their lives constantly worried about something. They find it remarkable that their friends can stay so cool.

Basically, it seems that to worry is quite normal; it is when you are worrying about worrying that you could be in trouble! The only real solution to over-anxiety is either to remove the source of the anxiety or to learn to cope with it so that it becomes less of a worry. Short-term use of tranquillizers may help people get over a bad patch, but they are no solution to longer-term anxieties. The anxiety will still be there, waiting to re-emerge, as soon as the opportunity arises.

What Is Insomnia?

We all have our own definitions of insomnia. For some, it is anything short of a full eight hours' sleep every night; for others, it is hardly sleeping a wink. Time and again, studies carried out in sleep laboratories have shown that we all sleep more than we think. People who say they have not slept in weeks all doze off at some time during the night. And many who claim to sleep badly at night catnap in an armchair during the afternoon and evening.

Sleep problems can take different forms. There are those who cannot get off to sleep at night and those who wake up in the small hours. Then there is the group who wake up with the dawn chorus and cannot get back to sleep again. Frequently, they lie awake worrying about the problems of the day. And these may be the people who are dosed up with tranquillizers during the day and sleeping pills to get them through the night. Modern sleeping pills do cater for the needs of people with different types of insomnia – some are better at getting sufferers off to sleep, others at getting them right through the night.

What Is Depression?

People frequently get anxiety and depression muddled up; doctors, too, have difficulty in defining exactly what they mean by each condition. Many depressed patients do suffer from anxiety and insomnia in addition to their underlying depression.

Most of us have, at some time, said 'I feel so depressed.' But in general we mean 'I'm fed up' rather than depressed. We have had a bad day, we did not get a job, we had a row with a friend. Such feelings can last hours, days or even weeks. But eventually something comes along to cheer us up and we certainly do not need drugs to get us out of our mood.

True depression does not disappear so easily. Doctors grade it, quite simply, mild, moderate or severe. Sometimes there is an obvious cause for the depression. The death of a husband or wife, a major illness in the family, the break-up of a marriage, perhaps; what the psychologists call a major life-event. In these cases, depression can take hold to such a degree that the sufferer cannot see a light at the end of the tunnel. Simply telling them they will get over it may not be enough and a course of antidepressant drugs may be necessary to get them through the difficult times until things do brighten up.

At other times the reason for the depression may be less obvious. Someone who seems to have coped with a bereavement or other crisis very well may lapse into depression several years later. Often, though, the cause of the depression remains a mystery. At its most severe, such depressives cannot function in daily life, they are interested in nothing; they become thin and listless and cannot sleep.

Antidepressant drugs, frequently in combination with psychiatric help, can relieve the depression. But little is known about the cause of the depression or the best form of treatment. Certainly, tranquillizers are of little use to such patients even though anxiety is a symptom of their condition. Between the white area of anxiety and the black of severe depression there are many shades of grey; and these are the most difficult patients to treat. These are the people who have some degree of anxiety and depression but who respond to neither group of drugs effectively.

Even with the group with the most easily defined type of depression, only 70 per cent respond to an antidepressant and over a third get better with a placebo. So it is hard to be sure just what the treatment is doing.

Who Needs Tranquillizers?

We all have our own ways of relaxing – some healthier than others. A hot bath, a good meal, an evening in front of the TV, a double gin. But what do we do when it does not work and the worries of the day seem to intrude on our every waking, and often sleeping, moment? Worries about work, worries about family, worries about the future.

In the short term, tranquillizers can be extremely effective in providing a breathing-space for someone whose worries have crowded in to such a degree that he simply cannot cope. But they should never be seen as a convenient alternative to sorting out what is at the root of those anxieties. There are no instant solutions to relieving anxiety. By the time they seek help from their doctor, some people will already have discussed their worries with family or friends; others will have been bottling them up, but many will not even have recognized what they are worried about, or indeed that anxiety is causing their mysterious aches and pains and feelings of unease.

A five-minute consultation with the doctor is hardly the time to unbottle anxieties which have been mounting for months and perhaps even years. So many doctors are prepared to hand out a prescription for a week's supply of tranquillizers on the understanding that patients will come back and start to discuss their anxieties in a longer interview. Unfortunately, some doctors then still take the easy way out and, instead of giving short-term prescriptions for tranquillizers accompanied by discussion of the patient's problems, prescribe initially for a month and then another and another . . . Before long the patient is well and truly hooked. Months turn into years; the anxieties may or may not have gone away but the tranquillizers are there to stay. A survey of tranquillizer users carried out by the *That's Life* programme in 1984 showed that over 90 per cent of respondents had taken the drugs for periods of four months or more – the duration recognized by the medical profession as the longest time tranquillizers should be used.

Nearly six years ago, in April 1980, one of the advisory committees to the DHSS, the Committee on the Review of Medicines, recommended that tranquillizers should not be used for periods of more than four months and sleeping pills for no longer than two to three weeks. This is because after those periods the body becomes tolerant to the effects of the drugs. They no longer work properly in relieving anxiety or insomnia, yet people may become addicted to them. Many doctors believe that even these periods are too long and that tranquillizers should only be taken in times of severe stress. After all, tranquillizers are not like antibiotics – you do not have to complete the course of treatment for them to work. Tranquillizers may be much better taken on a one-off basis when overwhelming feelings of anxiety overtake you, not religiously three times a day.

Bill started taking tranquillizers after his wife died. Her death had come as a big shock and Bill found it hard to carry on without her. The tranquillizers seemed to dull the pain of his bereavement and also helped him to sleep better.

Two years after his wife's death, Bill saw a TV programme which described some of the dangers of long-term use of sleeping pills and tranquillizers.

'I didn't like the idea of becoming addicted to the tranquillizers, and they mentioned my drug in particular by name. I asked the doctor if I should stop taking them and he said I was on such a small amount it didn't really matter,' said Bill.

But he decided to give up the drugs and had no trouble coming off them. He hasn't entirely got over his wife's death but he has found that he can now carry on his life without drugs.

Angela started taking tranquillizers because of her phobia. At one time she could hardly venture out of her house in case she had a panic attack.

She decided to contact her doctor after one particularly distressing episode. She was going to a company dinner with her husband, but no sooner had she got on the coach than she found herself too terrified to continue. Greatly embarrassed, she and her husband had to leave the coach and could not go to the dinner.

Angela was prescribed a tranquillizer so that if she felt a panic attack might occur she could calm herself.

'Knowing that I have the drugs has been a great confidence-booster,' said Angela. 'I don't take the drugs every day or even every week. But if I am going to something which I find rather worrying I take a tablet before I go out.'

Thanks to the drugs, Angela can hold down a job, take her children to school – and go to company dinners with her husband.

'I suppose I could try and do without them, but I don't want the phobia to come back so I'd prefer to be on the safe side.'

Who Needs Sleeping Pills?

Sleeping pills are used by a very diverse group of people and while there has been a small but steady decline in the number of prescriptions handed out for tranquillizers each year, prescriptions for sleeping pills have continued to hover around the seventeen million mark.

They are used by a range of people who, for one reason or another, find it hard to get a good night's sleep. The travelling salesman who rarely sleeps in the same bed on consecutive nights, the long-distance lorry driver who frequently sleeps in his cab or at roadside cafés, the shift-worker who works at night and tries to sleep during the day, the international executive who spends long periods in aeroplanes, crossing time zones and, not least, the men or women who sleep in their own beds in their own homes but simply cannot sleep.

Again, intermittent use of sleeping pills can work wonders for these groups of people but probably the most difficult to sort out will be those where there is no obvious cause of the insomnia.

A nurse or policeman on night duty may need sleeping pills for a few days at a time but will quickly revert to normal sleeping patterns once they get back to day duty. It is worrying to think of lorry drivers driving with the remains of sleeping pills in their blood but they too will probably only need them for short periods, and will be able to stop taking them when they return home; the same goes for the international traveller.

Many doctors will prescribe sleeping pills for intermittent uses such as these, just as they will give drugs for a couple of nights to try and re-establish a sleeping pattern in someone who is having trouble sleeping at home.

There are fifteen benzodiazepines promoted as sleeping pills on the market, though only three are prescribable on the NHS. All these drugs carry warnings about drinking alcohol or handling machinery while taking them, and experts recommend that doctors prescribe the shorter-acting sleeping pills which are less likely to produce hangover effects in the morning.

Nevertheless, many doctors are worried about the number of people who do drive or handle dangerous machinery while under the influence of sleeping pills or tranquillizers. One study carried out in Tayside to identify problem drinkers discovered a worryingly high proportion of drivers on the roads who had used both sleeping pills and alcohol. And studies carried out at Leeds University have shown that people on most benzodiazepines have significantly slower reactions compared to those who do not take them.

Jo is a nurse and regularly works night shifts, which means she comes off duty at 8.15 a.m. Just when the woman in the flat next door has her washing machine on and is starting the housework, Jo is trying to get off to sleep for the day.

'I know that life around me can't come to a standstill when I'm trying to sleep. But sometimes it seems that all I can hear is the vacuum cleaner one side, children screaming the other side, and the lawnmower going outside in the garden,' said Jo.

She used to take sleeping pills to help her get off to sleep and shut out the noises all around her. She would do a week of 'nights', during which she took sleeping pills. Then she got back to her normal sleeping pattern for three weeks of day duties.

'I didn't become addicted to them, but I found that I used to feel sleepy and hung over when I woke up. I just didn't feel right, so I stopped using them. I just stick to a milky drink now to try and get me off to sleep when I get in in the morning.'

How Do Sleeping Pills and Tranquillizers Work?

In spite of the fact that some benzodiazepines are recommended for the treatment of anxiety and others for insomnia, the whole family of drugs appears to work through the same mechanism. Precise details are still being worked out, but it appears that the benzodiazepines act on the area of the brain which handles our emotions; it is called the limbic system.

When we get anxious or excited the limbic system stimulates other areas of the brain so that we remain alert and ready for action. So that we do not live in a permanent state of frenetic activity the limbic system also contains a chemical to dampen things down and help us to relax. This has the impressive title of gamma amino butyric acid or GABA for short. Like other parts of the body, the limbic system can get it wrong and it seems that some people are not very good at activating their GABA and so they find it difficult to relax or sleep. This is where the benzodiazepines come in.

They stimulate GABA into action and thus have a calming effect. No one is sure whether people who suffer from anxiety are low in GABA and therefore find it hard to relax or whether there is a second chemical, similar to benzodiazepines, which boosts the effects of GABA and is missing in people who are over-anxious. No such natural relaxant has been found. But since a receptor has been found to which the benzodiazepine molecule binds, scientists have a shrewd idea that such natural tranquillizers do exist. Why otherwise would nature have provided a receptor? – not just for drug manufacturers to make use of, that's for sure.

Scientists have a lot to learn about chemicals in the brain. It is only ten years since they got to grips with the body's natural pain-killers, the endorphins. But if they find the body's natural benzodiazepines they will be able to boost them instead of having to replace them with drugs in people where there is a malfunction.

What's Wrong with Taking Tranquillizers?

Tranquillizers remain an extremely useful group of drugs. In the short term, taken for a few weeks to get someone through a bad patch while they work out a solution to their problems or, taken only once or twice a month in times of severe stress, tranquillizers can be highly effective. But problems, whether at work or at home, rarely just go away. Positive action needs to be taken either to remove or cope with them – and tranquillizers cannot do that.

Most people, when they first take benzodiazepine, get a feeling of calmness and a blurring of the senses, often within a few hours of the first tablet. Their problems do not go away, they simply appear less important. Is not that just what benzodiazepines are meant to do? And what is the harm in continuing to take them? There is good evidence that people do become addicted to benzo-diazepines and have unpleasant side-effects when they try to stop taking them. But for many people the idea of feeling anxious and upset if they stop taking their drugs seems far worse than being addicted to them. There is as yet little strong evidence of actual physical or mental damage from long-term use of benzodiazepines.

Brain scans from people taking such drugs have shown some abnormalities but experts are unsure just how important these are or whether they are reversible. There is little doubt that people taking tranquillizers and sleeping pills find it harder to concen-trate and remember things; their reactions are slowed. But for many people these facts are still not enough to convince them to try and give up. Often it is only possible to understand the effect the drugs were having after you have stopped taking them. And simply assuring people that they will feel so much better when they have given up may not be enough to entice them through the often difficult withdrawal phase.

Sometimes tranquillizer users are aware of changes in the way they handle life while they are taking the drugs. They feel they are somehow 'out of step' with other people. As with a transatlantic phone call, they are aware of slight pauses in their responses. Close friends and family get used to the change and they slip into a way of treating their tranquillized friends as slightly invalid –

they make allowances. Only outsiders are aware that something is 'different'.

None of us likes to think we are addicted to something – addiction is for junkies. How many smokers do you know who say they could give up any time if they really wanted? Or heavy drinkers who only drink to be 'sociable'. Addiction to tranquillizers does not happen overnight. Four to six months seems to be the cut-off point; after a year of taking them, one in five people will experience withdrawal symptoms when they try to give up. But that does not mean you will be all right if you only take them for three months and twenty-nine days. Sleeping pills and tranquillizers should be seen as a helping hand, never as a crutch.

Addiction to Tranquillizers and Sleeping Pills

It was around ten years ago that the first isolated reports trickled through describing withdrawal reactions experienced by people trying to give up benzodiazepines. As early as 1961, a year after the first of this group of drugs came on to the market, there was a report of withdrawal reactions which occurred after large doses of tranquillizer were taken. But such was the euphoria amongst doctors and their patients over the new 'happy pills' which appeared far safer than anything previously available for anxiety and insomnia, that the first warning went largely unnoticed.

No drug suits everyone and the early reports of unpleasant withdrawal problems were put down to the idiosyncrasies of a few people's responses. You do not abandon an important heart drug because a few people experience a loss of libido nor a useful arthritis drug because some patients suffer stomach problems. You simply find a more appropriate form of treatment for those who have problems and leave well alone those patients who are happy with their medication.

In addition, people who suffer most from anxiety tend to figure high on the neuroticism scales of psychologists' personality tests and many of the withdrawal reactions were put down either to 'neuroticism' or to a return of the anxiety for which the patients had been taking the drugs in the first place. Frequently, the only answer seemed to be to go back to the tranquillizers.

But by the beginning of this decade, the writing was on the wall. In 1980 the Committee on the Review of Medicines (CRM) recommended that people should only use tranquillizers and sleeping pills for short periods of time. There was no massive rush to pull patients off treatment but as more and more patients tried to stop their benzodiazepines in response to the CRM recommendation, the trickle of cases of withdrawal problems turned into a flood.

A study carried out by Nottingham doctors first reported at a scientific meeting and later published in the *Lancet* proved to be a turning-point. It concerned forty patients who had taken one of two commonly used tranquillizers regularly for an average of three and a half years. Their drugs were stopped and half the patients were given an alternative form of medication – a drug used to slow the heartbeat and reduce blood pressure – and the other half were given a placebo.

The trial was to last two weeks but, before it was over, eighteen of the patients – or nearly half – had dropped out of the study and returned to their tranquillizers because of withdrawal symptoms. The most common problems were extreme dysphoria and an impaired perception of movement. In other words, they were uncoordinated and felt miserable. Muscle-twitching, headaches, noise disturbance and retching and vomiting were also common withdrawal symptoms. Nearly half the patients experienced two or more of these symptoms and well over half had trouble sleeping.

The patients who were shifted from their tranquillizer to the heart drug suffered slightly fewer withdrawal problems than those on placebos. And, subsequently, this drug, a beta-blocker called propranolol, has been used widely both as an alternative to tranquillizers in the relief of acute anxiety and in providing a helping hand to patients trying to give up benzodiazepines. The people who suffered most were those whose blood levels of tranquillizer and its metabolites fell fastest. When levels fell more slowly withdrawal symptoms were less of a problem.

The Nottingham study seemed to open the floodgates. Paper after paper published in the academic research journals reported similar findings. One of these, published in the British Medical

Journal six months after the Nottingham paper came from two psychiatrists at the Institute of Psychiatry in London. They reported withdrawal symptoms in all sixteen patients they studied who had been on normal doses of benzodiazepines for long periods. Withdrawal of their drugs was slow; even so, all the patients reported symptoms of anxiety and tension, agitation and restlessness and sleep disturbance during the withdrawal phase.

The worst symptoms occurred between three and seven days after treatment was stopped and continued for two to four weeks. The doctors concluded that this group of drugs should not be given as regular daily treatment for chronic anxiety and pointed out that thousands of people were probably at risk, since an estimated 2 per cent of the adult population were thought to be on long-term benzodiazepines at that time.

How was it that so many people could be taking these drugs for such long periods? The repeat-prescription system used to a greater or lesser degree by virtually all GPs has been blamed for a high proportion of the patients left taking tranquillizers for ten, even twenty years. Between a quarter and a third of all prescriptions are handed out without the patient even seeing a doctor. Of course, where patients are on long-term therapy for a chronic condition, repeat prescribing makes a lot of sense.

People do not want to hang around in the waiting-room for a thirty-second consultation designed solely to get the doctor's signature on a prescription. And the doctor would prefer to spend even that short amount of time with another patient whose problems require a longer consultation. How much easier it is for the patient to make his request in writing or in person to the receptionist at the surgery who can arrange for a prescription to be ready the next day. No delay getting an appointment, no lengthy wait in the surgery, no unnecessary consultation.

Yet some doctors have abandoned the repeat-prescription system because it is so easily abused both by themselves and by their patients. Even someone on the most straightforward treatment with no obvious signs of problems should see the doctor from time to time and not rely solely on repeat prescriptions. After all, the patient, however well he may know his condition, is not a doctor and may fail to notice subtle changes in his condition which require attention.

Once high blood pressure is diagnosed, for example, many patients will need to take drugs to reduce it for the rest of their lives. When the appropriate dose is worked out there may not be any need to change the schedule for years but that does not mean there is no need for regular checks on pressure to make sure that everything is in order. The same goes for the asthmatic; his drugs may suit him well and his asthma may seem well controlled but basic lung function tests should be carried out in the surgery at regular intervals to make sure that all is well. Side-effects also need to be checked regularly in patients on long-term treatment. Patients come to accept many of their side-effects, even though alternative drugs exist which might suit them better. How is the doctor to judge unless she talks to her patient regularly?

No one should be tapped into the repeat-prescription system for tranquillizers or sleeping pills. New prescriptions for these drugs should be part of a programme of treatment, with the drugs merely 'tiding the patient over' until the next visit to the doctor, a week or so later. And even patients who have been taking such drugs for long periods and do not, at present, wish to stop them should be seeing their doctor regularly to check their progress and work out the best time to cut down and eventually stop taking them. If you simply turn up at the surgery every few months for a prescription for benzodiazepines you are not being treated for anxiety or insomnia, you are being conveniently forgotten.

Coming to terms with the underlying causes of anxiety or insomnia is not easy for the patient or for the doctor. But simply to keep taking the tablets without even seeing the doctor is to get second-class treatment. Equally, if you go to the doctor for endless prescriptions for tranquillizers without any proper discussion of the underlying problem you are being short-changed. A consultation which involves no more than the handing over of a prescription is no different from asking for the prescription at reception. A decision to reduce the dose and eventually to give up can come only after several lengthy consultations and with a lot of support from the doctor, your family and your friends. It cannot be accomplished in a meeting with your GP lasting only a few minutes.

Anne took tranquillizers for only three months and got no benefit from them at all. She had been complaining of mysterious aches and pains and sickness. Her doctor, unsure of what was wrong, prescribed tranquillizers.

'No one believed that there was something physically wrong with me. One day I started vomiting blood; I had been losing weight and I was frightened. I rang the hospital and they told me to come straight down. They found three large stomach ulcers. Later I saw a psychiatrist and he said there was nothing mentally wrong with me but my frustration at not being taken seriously almost certainly made my symptoms worse.'

Anne started to come off her tranquillizers and immediately experienced severe withdrawal symptoms – anxiety, palpitations, visual disturbances and unsteadiness; she kept bumping into things.

Eventually the withdrawal symptoms got better and she started taking an interest in life once more. In particular, she was now able to give her two daughters and her son more attention. Today, she never drinks coffee or alcohol and tries to avoid chocolate, since these can trigger withdrawal symptoms again. When she is anxious she still smokes; now she is trying to give up that too.

Margaret was only 19 when she was first prescribed a sleeping pill because she was 'going through a bad patch'. Prescription followed prescription and Margaret went through the range of sleeping pills, tranquillizers and antidepressants. It was only ater her second child was born that she was transferred on to the benzodiazepine group of drugs.

After more than 25 years of taking a variety of different drugs, Margaret went 'cold turkey'.

'I suddenly realized that it seemed that I always felt unwell and I decided to stop taking the drugs,' she said.

For two years after stopping her drugs Margaret 'went through hell'. She experienced a wide range of withdrawal symptoms from anxiety to insomnia, rage and misery, unsteadiness, nausea and feelings of unreality. Finally the curtain began to lift.

'For the first time in years I could see colours properly. I found the sky was so blue and grass so green. I was able to start doing some of the things I hadn't been able to do for years, like play the piano. The other day my daughter said to me, "You're different, you're not the mum I grew up with." I think that says it all.'

Susie is still trying to stop taking tranquillizers. They were first prescribed for panic attacks.

'I was convinced that either my children or I were going to be killed; each time I read of a murder I was sure it was going to happen to me. I would sit at the window and watch my children playing. I wouldn't let them out of my sight,' she said.

The drugs didn't stop her from panicking and Susie was worried about what they were doing to her health, so she decided to try to stop taking them. Each time she reduced the dose she experienced withdrawal symptoms, mainly of anger and rage.

'My children would come in from school and try and hug me. But I could not bear them to touch me. I love them dearly and the only time I could tell them was when they were asleep and I sat on the end of their bed and wept.'

The withdrawal effects are not so bad now. Susie still gets panicky, but at least she feels she can be a proper mother to her children and take an interest in life once more.

Coming off Benzodiazepines

It would be cruel to force someone to stop taking tranquillizers or sleeping pills if they did not feel ready. To succeed in stopping these drugs requires similar determination to stopping smoking. You cannot be half-hearted about it and you must want to stop taking them.

Fortunately, the first steps towards being an ex-tranquillizer user are slower than those to being an ex-smoker. Smokers are advised to give up completely from day one rather than to cut down and slowly reduce their habit. Benzodiazepines should be cut out slowly in order to minimize withdrawal effects. But in neither case should a slip-up – a couple of cigarettes or a return to a higher dose of drug – be seen as total failure. Begin again and persevere.

Although withdrawal symptoms can be unpleasant and some studies have shown very high incidences of side-effects, it is thought that over half of long-term users could stop their drugs without withdrawal problems. It has been suggested that people who have particularly dependent or passive natures are most prone to withdrawal problems but these are common traits in most patients who suffer from anxiety and insomnia.

Just how slowly you need to reduce the dose of your drugs should be discussed with your doctor. If you are on high doses then your withdrawal will probably need to be very gradual indeed. Some doctors recommend a quicker withdrawal because they believe that a very slow reduction prolongs the agony. A period of eight to ten weeks is favoured by many doctors but it is vital to discuss this with the doctor. You will also need the support of your family and friends so they should be included in the discussion. They do not need to know every detail but they may need to be a little more patient than usual and they may be able to help take you out of yourself if you are feeling unwell.

Although today's tranquillizer users are generally encouraged to take the shorter-acting drugs in the benzodiazepine family because they are less likely to cause side-effects, current thinking is to switch people planning to give up to the longer-acting drugs such as diazepam, just before the programme begins. This is because it generally takes longer for withdrawal effects to show themselves with the longer-acting drugs because levels in the blood are reduced more slowly. Instead of symptoms appearing within the first few days of stopping the drugs, they may not occur until after a week or so, by which time the patient may feel more able to cope with them.

Throughout the eight weeks or so of the withdrawal period, the dose is reduced only very slowly and, if withdrawal reactions do begin, it is quite possible to increase the dose of the benzodiazepine again for a few weeks until the patient feels on a more even keel. The important thing is not to rush the process. Once you have made up your mind to stop taking the drugs it does not have to happen overnight. You can leave it open-ended; just reduce the dose bit by bit and see when you are ready to stop. Some people continue on a tiny dose of benzodiazepine long after their bodies have ceased to need it. It does no harm and although it is scarcely more than a placebo it should not be seen as a failure.

For some people, the big breakthrough may come when they stop taking their tranquillizer every day. Although they may still be taking the same dose, spread over two days instead of one, it is the break from the daily routine which is crucial. The crutch is knocked away. No matter if it takes months; it is better to break the habit slowly and effectively so that you do not drift back on to the drugs later on.

Joining a Group

Many people do find it easier to give up their tranquillizers or sleeping pills with support from other people who have already given up or are in the process of doing so. Talking to others who know what it is like – the highs and lows, the goals to aim for and the pitfalls to avoid – has helped thousands of slimmers to stick to diets and smokers to give up cigarettes. And these group sessions are now being used successfully by people trying to get off benzodiazepines.

The largest of these organizations is called Tranx, which was started by Joan Jerome, herself a former tranquillizer user. Based in Harrow, the organization now has between twenty and thirty groups set up around the country to provide support for people trying to give up these drugs. The Harrow centre alone gets up to 600 inquiries a week.

Anyone who wishes to join first has to fill in a questionnaire detailing the drugs they are taking. The staff at the centre are not medically qualified although they do have extensive medical back-up from acknowledged experts in the field. Members are then sent information about how to reduce the dosage of their drugs and are encouraged to attend the centre for support meetings. At these, members discuss what has been happening to them; their good days and their bad, and express any anxieties or depression. Frequently they can be reassured that certain difficulties they are experiencing will pass or that withdrawal symptoms are to be expected and not a sign of something more serious.

The emphasis is on slow withdrawal of drugs and steady recovery – far longer than the ten to twelve weeks recommended by many doctors. The emphasis is on patients deciding for themselves when they feel ready to stop the drugs altogether and doses are reduced only very gradually. How long people attend centres like that at Harrow varies enormously. Some people go to the centre several times a week for many weeks, others may only go once or twice. Merely to know that support is there is sufficient for many people to go away and come off their drugs on their own.

On the whole, groups like Tranx deal with people who have been unable to get the support they feel they need from their own doctor, family or friends in stopping their tranquillizers or sleeping pills. In spite of the vast amounts of publicity surrounding the hazards of long-term use of benzodiazepines there are some doctors who still believe that their patients should remain on their drugs in spite of their expressed desire to stop taking them. Or they do not want to be troubled with getting their patient through the withdrawal phase. For these people, support groups such as Tranx may be the only practical option.

In general, Joan Jerome has found that the best results from her support groups tend to be for people who either attend the centre or are in regular contact, though there is no question of insisting that members attend. Groups other than Tranx do exist around the country, some run by health professionals, others by former drug users. The best way to find out if there is a support group in your area is to contact your local community health council which generally has a record of health groups and clinics in the area.

Joy couldn't bear even to sit in on the meetings of the support group when she first joined. She ran out of the room each time other members of the group described their withdrawal symptoms. 'I had been taking tranquillizers and antidepressants since I was 15. By the time I was in my early thirties it seemed as though my life was over; my marriage had broken up and I was suicidal,' she said.

When Joy started going to the group she relied on daily phone calls from other members to keep her spirits up and help her stay off the drugs.

'I don't know what I would have done without the group. At last I found that I wasn't odd and that other people were experiencing the same problems as me. The support I have got has been very important to me.'

Michael read in his local newspaper about a support group for people trying to get off tranquillizers and sleeping pills. He had been taking benzodiazepines on and off for twelve years, but had received little support from his GP when he said that he would like to stop taking drugs.

'I have found the support group very helpful. When you're having withdrawal symptoms you can tell other people in the group and they know what it's like. I don't think I could get off the drugs without the group.'

Alternatives to Drugs

Counselling

It is thought that at least one in three people who go to their doctors are troubled in mind rather than in body. This is not to suggest that these people are insane, but many are unaware that their physical symptoms – odd aches and pains, tiredness and lethargy – are clues to underlying emotional problems. A doctor's detective work does not stop at piecing together the physical picture, it must also interpret the vague signals of mental unease.

Diagnosing a physical illness is generally a lot easier than getting to grips with an emotional problem. Physical examination combined with laboratory and other tests can rule out many of the options for physical illness and give a good idea of what is wrong. But mental and emotional problems rarely show up in laboratory tests and require lengthy questioning on the part of the doctor and a desire to co-operate from the patient.

Medical students are taught these basic consultation skills during their training but, while some doctors find it relatively easy to talk at length with their patients about their worries, others find it much more difficult. They may be very good at recognizing the early symptoms of a rare physical disease but find it much harder to talk about emotional problems with patients who are embarrassed and unwilling to expose their emotional wounds.

Some of us are better at listening to the woes of our friends than others. How many times have we found ourselves saying, 'I can really talk to her', when we have found it impossible to bare our souls to other friends who are just as dear to us. So it is with doctors; some are easy listeners and good advisers, others less so. Their impartiality confers both advantages and disadvantages. On the one hand we may find it harder to tell our troubles to someone we do not know but, on the other, the impersonal nature of the consultation in the surgery may help us to express thoughts we would not be able to otherwise.

The long tradition of the doctor as a father-figure who can help in times of trouble can also help some patients, although the all-powerful, almost god-like, figure of the doctor who knows best is fortunately disappearing. Everyone makes mistakes and doctors are no exception. So any discussion of emotional or personal problems should not centre around what the doctor would do if she were in the same situation but should enable the patient to consider the options available and come to his or her own decision.

If we simply want an opinion on what we should do, we can go to our friends or relatives. They tend to be full of advice. Frequently, we know deep down the best way forward but need someone to put the options in front of us and prod us into deciding. As one GP recently put it 'I know when I've helped someone with an emotional dilemma. They leave the surgery and tell their friends I was not much use – they made up their own mind after all.'

This listening role has been part and parcel of the relationship between doctor and patient for generations. Before the advent of modern forms of treatment it was frequently all that was available. She might not know what was wrong with his patient or be able to treat him, but at least the doctor could lend a friendly ear. And it frequently had to suffice for physical as well as emotional illness.

But as science has taken over in the surgery, both doctor and patient have come to rely on what drugs and other forms of treatment have to offer in both physical and emotional illness. We have already seen how the barbiturates took over from the sympathetic ear for the anxious and sleepless during the Fifties and Sixties and how the benzodiazepines took over from them. Now, as the dangers of long-term use of these drugs are recognized, the story has come full circle and we are turning once again to the listening rather than the prescribing skills of the doctor.

They have become rusty in the intervening years and they have taken on a new name, counselling – and they are in short supply. In its strictest sense, counselling is neither treatment nor, simply, advice and support. It involves helping people to make decisions by prodding them into examining their feelings more deeply than if they were on their own. But the word 'counselling' has taken on a much more general meaning, so it is probably easier to look at it in its broadest sense, in the forms in which we, as patients, may encounter it.

Some doctors feel that 'counselling' is part of their daily job and comes into every consultation. But at five minutes per person there is not much time for winkling out the causes of anxiety during an ordinary visit with the doctor. Others accept that they have neither the time nor the talent to talk at length with patients about emotional problems. And they either turn these patients over to someone more skilled in this area or, sadly, they wash their hands of the problem and reach for the prescription-pad. A few run 'listening clinics' when time is specially set aside for people who have emotional problems and need a longer than average consultation.

What is counselling?

Counselling happens at many levels, and basically equates with making the patient feel that someone is taking an interest in them and trying to help. Those most interested in counselling are determined that it should not be seen as some mysterious ability practised by a few which enables the rest to ignore the whole idea of talking to patients.

Counselling can begin from the moment the patient makes an appointment or goes to the surgery. The receptionist can help the patient feel important and not just another name to add to the long list for the Monday morning surgery. By responding to feelers which the anxious patient puts out, whether they concern the weather or the colour of the waiting-room, the receptionist can help in the long process of making the patient feel at ease and ready to unburden his problems. The same goes for other members of the primary health-care team – the practice nurse, the health visitor and any other people the patient may meet at the surgery or during visits at home. The worst thing of all would be for patients to be pigeon-holed for the counsellor and ignored by other members of the team.

People involved in counselling find it hard to define exactly what the process involves. The ultimate aim is to help the patient cope with his anxieties, either by changing his lifestyle to avoid those things which make him most anxious or by learning to deal with them better. Clinical psychologists concentrate more on modifying particular aspects of behaviour, which may be worrying the patient or upsetting his family, and thus bringing stress back on to himself; other counsellors concentrate on encouraging patients to develop skills which may have been buried and can give them the strength to deal with their problems; others simply listen and help patients to feel that someone cares.

No particular brand of counselling is right for every patient who comes into the surgery and says, 'I don't know what's wrong – I just seem to be worried all the time.' In some cases they need to be encouraged to identify their skills and develop them and in others they may need to get into perspective areas where they simply over-react.

This brief description is an over-simplification of the many and varied roads which counselling can take. And just as the form of the counselling can vary so does the duration.

Counselling sessions generally last for about an hour but some people may find it hard to unburden themselves to a comparative stranger for such a length of time, and may prefer to start with short discussions and build up to a longer meeting. Some patients feel better after only a few sessions and go away more able to cope with their problems, others may need many months of counselling before they can feel the benefit.

Some practices refer patients for counselling to the doctor in the group who seems best at it; others refer patients to outside counsellors and a very few pay a counsellor as a member of the health team and make the service a part of the NHS. Outside counsellors can charge anything from £6 to £20 per session.

The British Association for Counselling (BAC) was set up in 1977 and has over 2000 individual members and 130 organizational members. It defines the task of counselling as giving a client the opportunity to explore, discover and clarify ways of living more resourcefully and towards greater well-being. Many of the counsellors already employed directly or indirectly by general practitioners are members of the BAC, which is pressing for more widespread recognition of the importance of counselling in general practice by trying to get it available on the NHS. At present, GPs who employ counsellors and do not charge patients either pay the counsellors out of general-practice funds or reclaim the salary by calling the counsellor secretarial or clerical staff for which they can be reimbursed officially. The only other alternative is to charge patients.

If you are looking for a counsellor and your GP cannot recommend one, you should try and ensure that your counsellor has been accredited to the BAC. This means that his or her training or experience will have been checked by the Association to ensure it is sufficient to enable the counsellor to do a worthwhile job. No doubt there are good counsellors outside the BAC but, as with any unregistered health profession, it is inevitable that there are some people practising without qualifications who are unsuitable. And until counselling becomes a recognized part of health care this is likely to remain the case.

Alongside counsellors working in general practice are the more specialist counsellors working for the National Marriage Guidance Council (NMGC). A high proportion of anxieties which take patients to the doctor's surgery in search of help stem from trouble at home within the family. Problems within a marriage, difficulties with children and misunderstandings with in-laws all take their toll on our overall sense of well-being. The Council is finding that people nowadays tend to seek help earlier, when problems first start to arise, rather than when a marriage is on the rocks and reconciliation at its most difficult. Already, some marriage-guidance counsellors do have links with general practices and the NMGC is keen to extend these.

Does counselling work?

It is very difficult to quantify the effectiveness of counselling and other therapies for emotional problems. You can measure the effectiveness of different treatments of cancer in terms of survival rates; the same goes for certain types of surgery. And you can test whether drugs have worked by comparing their effectiveness with what happens when no drugs are given. But such things as feelings of well-being and ability to cope with life are highly subjective and do not lend themselves easily to statistical analysis.

Assessments of the effectiveness of counselling have, until now, depended upon whether it has influenced the number of prescriptions for tranquillizers and sleeping pills. Surely, if counselling works, people will need fewer of these drugs and, after the initial intensive period of counselling, they will be less likely to go to their doctor with anxiety-related problems? Well . . . yes and no.

Studies have yielded mixed results. Not all report a reduction in drug usage. The same goes for the number of consultations with a doctor. Many of the studies only followed up the patients for a few months after counselling and others showed that even where there was a fall in the need for medical help this was sometimes reversed when the patients were checked several months or a year or so later. In one of the most recent studies, involving a six-year follow-up, there were marked falls in the number of both prescriptions and consultations, but psychologists could not be sure whether this was simply as a result of the natural course of the patients' illnesses. After all, some patients do get better without help from drugs or other therapy. The particular crises pass or they adapt on their own to the stresses in their lives.

Some doctors believe that we will have to wait longer to see the advantages of counselling and that the number of prescriptions, or of consultations, is the wrong criterion for measuring the effectiveness of treatment. Instead, they feel that long-term death and illness statistics will reflect the value of counselling. There is already some evidence that people who feel good about themselves are better at coping with common illnesses and with even more serious diseases such as cancer. So it could be that the reduced anxiety and greater sense of well-being conferred by counselling may help people live longer, happier lives.

At present this is conjectural and it will be some years before any trends in statistics can show the benefits of counselling. Not everyone will be helped by this approach to treatment. Some people find it hard to express their thoughts and feelings even with the most patient of listeners. Their fears and worries are likely to remain bottled up, and neither drugs nor counselling will be able to solve them. Other forms of therapy are available, though these too may not be available on the NHS and, like counselling, they do not have all the answers.

The divide between counselling and psychotherapy is frequently a hazy one. At its most specific, the difference between the two forms of therapy is that counselling tends to be a listening therapy whereas psychotherapy is much more interactive, with the psychotherapist contributing more of his or her own thoughts about the client's problems. Both partners contribute to the relationship. But just as counselling can take many forms, so can psychotherapy. Some people conduct a more interactive form of counselling, while some psychotherapists' approach is more akin to counselling. There is a grey area between the two forms of therapy where there is considerable overlap between the two approaches. The training of psychotherapists is generally more intensive than that for counsellors.

In some cases the psychotherapist is likely to take on more long-term therapy for people with more deep-rooted problems rather than those who are experiencing transient anxiety or stress problems. Again, some practices have access to a trained psychotherapist although you are likely to have to pay for sessions. Or, if you have difficulty in finding a qualified therapist, the British Association of Psychotherapists may be able to advise.

Coping with Anxiety

What happens when the counselling or psychotherapy stops? There are no time limits for how long people can continue with these sessions, but neither counsellors nor therapists see themselves simply as a long-term substitute for tranquillizers. They can help people make decisions on their immediate problems and come to terms with the long-standing difficulties which have made them over-anxious. But stress does not come in neat packages which can be unwrapped and sorted out every few years. It is a continuing process which may need daily – even hourly – intervention from us to keep it in check.

For some it may be enough simply to say, 'Stop, I've had enough', but others may need specific relaxation techniques to help them slow down and stop worrying. Yoga, massage, meditation and hypnosis all have their exponents. And the old image of relaxation classes of people lying on the floor doing breathing exercises is definitely outdated. No single method of relaxation is likely to work for everyone but three tried and tested methods are widely practised. Progressive relaxation involves tensing and relaxing small groups of muscles in the body one by one. The idea is to be able eventually to localize specific muscles which are tense and relax them. Another form of relaxation, called autogenic training, also involves relaxation of the limbs but this time uses a sort of self-hypnosis. The third method involves thinking about some particularly relaxing scene and picking out and focusing on the aspects of the picture that are most relaxing.

All of these methods of relaxation take some time to master – you do not just lie down one evening and learn to relax every set of muscles. A number of organizations, such as the Stress Foundation, produce leaflets, tapes and other information about relaxation, as well as running classes in the basic techniques. Some doctors also refer patients to relaxation therapists. But relaxation is for more than just those who have gone to their doctor because of anxiety.

Some of us seem intent on making life as difficult as possible for ourselves by building up our stress and anxiety to fever pitch. Many of us argue that we function at our best under pressure. But we do not have to leave everything until the last minute or insist on doing every last piece of work ourselves instead of delegating to others. Dealing with day-to-day stresses and anxieties should be a mix of coping and avoiding. Counselling, therapy, relaxation and tranquillizers all have their place, but so does having the common sense to realize when you have taken on too much . . . and saying so!

CHAPTER 8

Ask the Pharmacist

Long gone are the days when the pharmacist spent his days bent over pestle and mortar concocting medicines for the needy, with recipes for mysterious remedies handed down through genera- tions and jealously guarded from rival apothecaries. Today's pharmacists are taught how to manufacture medicines during their training but rarely have to put that knowledge to use during their everyday work in the chemist's shop. Those who look after medicines in hospitals are more likely to have to make up specific medicines – for cancer patients, for example – but the vast majority of medicines come ready-made in large packages direct from the manufacturer.

Yet the 25,000 pharmacists currently practising in Britain have all spent three years of intensive training to qualify for their degrees in pharmacy. They know vastly more about how medi- cines are made than doctors, and they are also taught more about how they work; they know less about the anatomy and physiology of the body and they are not taught how to diagnose illness. But they are well equipped to advise how to take medicines and to recognize unwanted effects of drugs when they arise. Over 70 per cent of trained pharmacists work in chemists' shops – so-called pharmacies. They deal with over a million prescriptions every day. The remaining 7000 working pharmacists in Britain work in hospitals, industry, education or government service.

It is expected that by 1987 nearly all drugs will arrive at the pharmacy pre-packed by drug firms, ready to be handed to patients. Even the current need to transfer medicines from the large bulk packs supplied by drug companies into the smaller individualized bottles of medicines which patients take home – a job for which highly trained pharmacists are vastly overquali- fied – will disappear. For years pharmacists have complained that they did not train for three years just so that they could fill bottles with medicines. Now even this function is disappearing.

In the autumn of 1983, an independent inquiry was set up to examine the present and future role of pharmacists in health care. It is expected that the government will assess these recommendations to decide how they may be implemented. The Nuffield Inquiry, as it was called, had no official status but does have DHSS blessing and no government likes to waste money training professional people only to see their original function eroded away. This is what has happened to pharmacists and it seems that they may be at the beginning of a new phase in their history when they come out from behind their pharmacy counters and offer a form of health care more complementary to that provided by doctors, health visitors and others working in the community.

If the professional role of the pharmacist is to be expanded, then it has been argued that pharmacists will have to stop selling everything from cosmetics to cuddly toys in their shops and return once more to dispensing drugs alone. But for many pharmacists, competing with other shops in the high street as well as the large retail chemists, the only way to make a living is to sell goods other than medicines and toiletries. Clearly, it will not be enough just to restore the professional role of the pharmacist and make him a fully paid-up member of the health-care team, he will have to make a decent living too.

Such a large-scale reorganization of pharmacists will take years to carry out. In the meantime, we are increasingly encouraged to 'ask the pharmacist' rather than bothering the doctor with minor complaints. How can our pharmacist help us? He may know all about how drugs work but can he answer day-to-day problems about our medicines?

What Can We Ask the Pharmacist?

At some time or another we have all asked the pharmacist what he would recommend for a tickly cough, an upset tummy or some stubborn spots. Sometimes it is not even the pharmacist whom we ask, but whoever is serving behind the counter. They may recommend a medicine they have heard the pharmacist suggest before or they may check with the pharmacist. But if you are unsure whether the assistant is competent to answer your query you can always ask to speak to the pharmacist personally. A pharmacist's course lasts three years but before he or she can practise as a qualified pharmacist they must do a 'pre-registration' year at the end of his or her course at university. At least six months of this period must be spent working with patients, either at a chemist's shop or in a hospital. These trainees know all about the drugs they are dispensing but they are less experienced at dealing with customers.

Sometimes the pharmacist will advise you to see your doctor because he feels that your illness needs to be properly checked, requiring possibly more than just a medicine which you can buy from the chemist. At other times he may sell you a simple remedy and advise you to see your doctor if the problem does not clear up in a few days. We have already seen how many patients unfortunately waste their own and their doctor's time by going to see her with a cough or cold which will clear up on its own in less than a week. Something for a sore throat or a cough may make you feel better in the meantime but these may be bought at the chemist, where they are frequently cheaper than a prescription. Many such remedies are no longer prescribable on the NHS and can only be obtained from the chemist. By going to the pharmacist first you may avoid a trip to the doctor and leave the latter with extra time to treat people with more serious illnesses which need more than a five-minute consultation.

Pharmacists can also help with drugs prescribed by the doctor. No one should leave the chemist's shop with medicines unless they are clear in their minds about how to take them; how many tablets to take, how often they should be taken, whether they should be taken at any particular time of day, with food or without, and how long to go on taking them.

Unfortunately, the label on the bottle rarely carries all this information. If your medicine comes in pre-packed containers straight from the drug company it is likely to carry more information than the average medicine bottle containing a limited supply of tablets, which only has to have the pharmacist's name and address, your name, the name of the drug and the date on which it was dispensed. The pharmacist can include details of dosage even if the doctor has not written these on the prescription. But we still get medicines with 'as before' or 'as directed' on the label – leaving it to us to remember the dose. This is not very helpful. We have already seen how hard it is to remember what the doctor says in surgery, and few of us take in details of doses and timing, often of more than one drug, at the first attempt.

If you cannot remember the instructions about your medicine when you get to the pharmacist, and the doctor did not write instructions on the prescription, ask the pharmacist to telephone the doctor for the information. He will have written in his notes how he intended the drug to be taken and can easily check. Better still, ask your doctor to write down the dose for you, preferably on the prescription, before you leave the surgery.

The pharmacist has no fewer than twenty-eight different warnings and pieces of advice which the Pharmaceutical Society recommends should be put on labels of bottles of medicines. They do not apply to all medicines, of course. But some medicines should carry advice as to whether they need to be taken with plenty of water or with food, on an empty stomach or at bedtime. Others can cause drowsiness or the patient should avoid alcohol during the course of treatment. All of these simple pieces of advice are important in helping the patient get the most from his medicine. But, all too frequently, they are left off and the hapless patient has to take his medicines as best he can.

As more drugs are supplied with information leaflets, it has been suggested that pharmacists could hand them out and go through them with patients. After all, it is the pharmacist who is the last professional 'port of call' for the patient before he takes his drugs, and information at this stage may have less chance of being forgotten.

Pharmacists are also in an excellent position to remind patients about side-effects they may experience while taking their medicine and to warn them not to buy over-the-counter drugs which might mix badly with their prescribed drugs. Drugs sold by the pharmacist fall into two categories; medicines that come on the 'general sales' list and which can also be sold at other shops such as supermarkets and newsagents, and pharmacy-only drugs that can be sold only under the supervision of a pharmacist and which are not therefore available in other shops.

In general terms, it is the more potent drugs which have to be sold under the supervision of a pharmacist, that is, drugs which need accompanying advice from some suitably qualified person about how they should be used. Thus many headache and indigestion products can be bought at supermarket or grocery stores but cough mixtures such as Benylin and Actifed can only be sold at chemists' shops where a qualified pharmacist is on hand. Even so, large quantities of pain-killers such as aspirin and paracetamol cannot be bought outside pharmacies. Thus, you can buy a small pack of aspirin containing up to twenty-five tablets at the grocer but larger packs must be bought at the chemist's. You can buy slightly more – up to thirty tablets – if the aspirin is in effervescent form, but more than that and you will have to go to the chemist. The object of these limits is to discourage people from taking large quantities, or more than the recommended dose of such drugs, though someone who was determined could of course buy several small packs of aspirin at different supermarkets.

In recent years there has been a trend towards allowing some drugs previously available only on prescription to be sold under the supervision of the pharmacist. Loperamide, sold as Arret for the treatment of diarrhoea, and ibuprofen, sold as Nurofen, are two recent examples. Both these drugs used to require a prescription; many arthritic patients have been and will continue to be prescribed ibuprofen by their doctors, generally under the brand name, Brufen. But now, patients can buy it for all forms of pain, including that linked to arthritis, direct from the chemist.

Both drugs had an excellent track record for safety and effectiveness and it was felt that they could be made more generally available. However, they can be bought only from a pharmacist since it may be important to advise patients of specific side-effects. Nurofen, for example, like many pain-killers of its type can cause stomach irritation to susceptible people, and so it is important for the pharmacist to check that someone wishing to buy the drug does not have stomach ulcers or dyspepsia.

Britain has been relatively strict about the drugs it has made more freely available. In some countries patients can buy more drugs from their pharmacist, without a doctor's prescription. And in many developing countries there is no prescription system at all. You can buy almost anything from the pharmacist provided you can afford to pay.

A number of drugs – including some antibiotics, allergy preparations and even the contraceptive pill – have been proposed to follow loperamide and ibuprofen off the prescription-pad and on to the pharmacy shelves. But such radical proposals are unlikely to be taken up at present.

Pharmacists, like doctors, vary in the amount of information they give to customers about both their prescribed drugs and the medicines they buy direct. But they are in an excellent position to notice side-effects which customers experience. For example, if one of their regular customers suddenly starts coming in to buy something for indigestion or constipation when they never previously required such medicines, the pharmacist may wonder whether these problems are side-effects of a new medicine which the customer has been prescribed. Not only can he advise the customer on drugs to buy which will not interfere with his other medicines, he can also suggest that the customer should go back to his doctor and ask whether he might have an alternative drug to avoid such side-effects.

At present the pharmacist cannot report side-effects which he notices amongst patients directly to the DHSS, but the Pharmaceutical Society is pressing for the yellow-card reporting scheme to be extended to pharmacists. Already, hospital pharmacists can fill in yellow cards for doctors to sign if they notice side-effects which they feel should be reported. But pharmacists working in shops can only advise their local doctor of side-effects and leave him to decide what action to take.

The pharmacists best suited to recognizing side-effects are those who have regular customers that they know well. Clearly, if a total stranger comes in asking for drugs for indigestion the pharmacist will have no idea whether this is a drug side-effect or a symptom often suffered by the patient. This is one reason why some pharmacists favour the idea of patients registering with them as they would with a doctor. But would a system of registration work? Should pharmacists keep records about their customers just like those of a doctor? Or would this mean an unnecessary duplication of information and long waits for the patient while the pharmacist consulted his records before dispensing prescriptions?

Registering with a Pharmacist

Some pharmacists who have a large number of regular customers already keep records about some of them – generally the elderly or those on long-term medication involving several different drugs. Such records take different forms, ranging from simple card indexes with the names of patients' drugs written on them, to fully computerized record systems. In some cases patients carry record cards of their own which can be cross-checked with those held in the pharmacy, so that if they get any drugs at another chemist's these can be written on the card and the files of their own pharmacist brought up to date, next time they go in.

By keeping records, pharmacists believe that they are better able to spot errors on prescriptions, pick up side-effects, and help patients avoid drugs which might interact with each other. Mistakes do occur on prescriptions; doctors, or receptionists writing repeat prescriptions for doctors to sign, can write down the wrong dose or frequency with which a drug should be taken. If the pharmacist is unfamiliar with what the patient was taking previously he may dispense the drug without realizing that the patient has been prescribed double, treble, even ten times his normal dose. Similarly, if he is unaware of other medications the patient is taking, he may not notice that a new medicine might interact badly with a drug already being taken. Remember that an estimated 5 per cent of hospital admissions and one in forty visits to the general practitioner are thought to be made necessary by adverse reactions to drugs.

One London pharmacist who has kept records of his customers' drugs carried out a survey of how many potential adverse reactions he spotted with the help of his record system. Cards were kept on the drugs taken by 1366 patients and, in the first three years in which the system operated, the pharmacist identified eighty-six potential reactions. In fifty-three of these cases the doctor changed the prescription when his attention was drawn to the potential problem and in a further fifteen cases patients were advised about how to reduce the risk of adverse reactions. During this time seventy-six errors on prescriptions were spotted, generally unintentional changes of the dose or strength of tablets.

Just how often doctors make serious errors over their

prescriptions is open to debate. If the pattern found in the London survey is typical of the rest of the country, then there could be some 300,000 similar potential adverse reactions in general practice each year. Some mistakes will be so obvious they will be easily picked up and avoided, others may not have harmful effects. But that still leaves a substantial core of mistakes with potentially serious outcomes for the patient. And more widespread systems of record-keeping amongst pharmacists could help reduce the risks for the patients. Record systems are all very well for the small-town, high-street pharmacist who knows his clients well. But what about people who rarely collect their prescription from the same chemist and live in cities? How is the pharmacist to keep track of what they are taking? There are two options: either patients could register with the pharmacist in their nearest high street or they, rather than their pharmacist, could keep records of the drugs they are taking.

The first option, registration with pharmacists, would create a massive upheaval in the present system of dispensing drugs. Its advantages would be that all pharmacists would know their customers and could keep a check on their drugs. The major disadvantage would be the inconvenience to patients who rarely collect their drugs from the same chemist and would, in future, be tied to their local pharmacy. Doubtless arrangements could be made in an emergency for patients to collect drugs from pharmacies miles from their homes, just as there are systems for people on holiday to see local doctors if they are taken ill. But, in general, people would have to become used to obtaining their drugs from the pharmacy to which they were allocated rather than the one most convenient on any particular day.

The alternative to this – patients carrying their own records – is already being investigated. One of the most interesting projects has been carried out in Cardiff where some 300 patients have been issued with a plastic key which fits on an ordinary key-ring. Each contains a microchip with coded details of the drugs the owner is taking, and can only be read when the key is fitted into the 'lock' on a central computer in the local pharmacy. The pharmacist can see at a glance the drugs which the patient is taking and can add information about new drugs or delete old, out-of-date information.

If such a system became used nationally, a patient could go into any chemist's shop in the country with a prescription, present his key to enable the pharmacist to check his drugs and have details of the new prescription added. Discrepancies over dosage compared with previous prescriptions could be checked and any possible drug interactions between prescribed drugs or between prescribed and bought drugs could be picked up. This sort of system is not as futuristic as it sounds. A similar idea, using a form of 'credit card' to store the information about drugs is already used in parts of Europe, and as more and more pharmacists invest in computers it would not be difficult to link the records into their own systems.

It would mean little or no inconvenience to the patient since it takes a very few minutes to link the key into the computer, add new information and dispense the drugs. Most people carry a batch of keys or a handful of credit cards so either format would fit easily into pockets or handbags. It would mean little extra work for the pharmacist and require no extra storage facilities as the pharmacist would not need to keep his own patient records. But it might mean more headaches for the doctor. Would the average GP take kindly to having more of his prescriptions questioned – as would inevitably happen? And how would pharmacists decide which were serious problems, necessitating a check with the doctor, and which were relatively trivial and easily corrected discrepancies in prescribing?

Pharmacists Talking to Doctors

No one likes their judgement questioned and doctors, more than most professionals, are not used to having their decisions queried. Links between GPs and their local pharmacists vary enormously and, like most working relationships, depend largely on the personalities of those involved.

Some doctors do not mind when the pharmacist rings them to check something they have written on a prescription, others cannot abide interference. Equally, some pharmacists can be very tactful when checking an incorrectly written dose or quantity of drugs, while for others it is a game of one-upmanship. But for many doctors it seems that they only hear from their local pharmacists when they have done something wrong. In some parts of the country, more enlightened pharmacists and doctors meet regularly on joint committees to iron out any problems. They can discuss individual cases and how drugs should be prescribed. Grievances are aired rather than bottled up.

There is also a move towards some pharmacists actually working in health centres. Patients collect their prescriptions and get them dispensed immediately by the resident pharmacist and his team. Often this works well; if there are any queries over drugs the pharmacist can pop into the doctor's office or pick up an internal phone and check it on the spot. Regular joint meetings enable all members of the health-care team to discuss any problems. And, because pharmacists regularly see the same patients, they get used to the drugs they are taking and can quickly spot any errors.

Inevitably, such systems have also seen their failures. One partner in the practice may be only to happy to talk to the pharmacist whenever problems arise, while other partners are less keen. Other local pharmacists may be unhappy as they see the bulk of local dispensing being handled by the pharmacist linked up to the health centre. No scheme, however sensible in theory, runs smoothly all the time. The medical profession is wary of pharmacists intruding too far on to its patch. In their 1984 Pharmacists' Charter and in their evidence to the Nuffield Inquiry, the pharmacists put up a strong case for taking on a greater role in the primary care of patients. And many of these proposals were met with hostility by the medical profession.

For example, it was suggested that pharmacists could extend their advisory role to patients to the extent of having their own consulting-rooms within their shops. Already many pharmacists have set aside a small section of the shop for discussing the taking of medicines with patients. Some pharmacists have taken this one step further and do provide a small consulting-room where patients can talk privately with the pharmacist. Some people believe this is taking the consulting process too far. After all, one of the reasons patients like to discuss their problems with the pharmacist is because of the informal nature of the discussions. Providing a consulting-room may make the patient feel uncomfortable and put the consultation on a similar level to that with the doctor, with whom the patient frequently finds it hard to communicate. In addition, some patients may feel conspicuous if they disappear into another room with the pharmacist. On the other hand a separate consulting-room or at least a small area in the shop set aside for advice does provide a greater degree of privacy for people wanting to discuss personal health problems.

Another of the pharmacists' proposals was that they should be able to carry out visits to the homes of elderly, or chronically sick patients. They argue that since it is they who know most about the drugs, it should be their place to make sure that housebound patients are taking their medicines correctly. After all, these people – who are frequently those most at risk from the adverse effects of drugs or interactions between different drugs – may get their information about using them second- or third-hand. The pharmacist may remind whoever picks up their medicines about dose, timing and other precautions but this information may not get passed on to the person who is actually going to take the drugs. By visiting them at home the pharmacist could check they were taking their medicines regularly, and storing them correctly.

A growing number of cancer patients are taking complicated combinations of drugs at home. Those fortunate enough to have access to specialist nursing facilities, such as the Macmillan or Marie Curie nurses, will find it easy to get their questions answered about doses of pain-killers and other drugs. But other patients may be less fortunate in getting speedy answers to pressing questions about the drugs they are taking and the pharmacist could provide an important line of information. Obviously, the introduction of the pharmacist into the health-care team visiting the elderly and chronically sick would have to be carried out with the greatest care. Conflicting information from too many different sources would be worse than no information at all. People could end up confused and frightened, not knowing whom to turn to.

In the past, pharmacists may not have been taught sufficient communication skills to enable them to carry out home visits and discuss drugs with patients. But as the emphasis in teaching curricula for pharmacists shifts towards better communication, pharmacists could become as adept at explaining about drugs to patients as nurses and health visitors are about other aspects of health education. The skills of the members of the health-care team should be seen as complementary rather than competitive.

Inevitably, there are doctors, and other health professionals, who see the pharmacists as a profession looking for a job. Their job behind the chemist's counter has been taken over by the high-technology drug companies so they are looking for work in front of the counter and out in the community. And if pharmacists are to take on a community health role how will they be paid? At present their income depends to some extent on sales of other consumer goods within their shops. In return for getting rid of some of the more dubious goods in their stores should they be paid for the advisory service which they are being encouraged to provide?

The way in which pharmacists are currently paid must be one of the most complicated in the world – only a handful of people truly understand it. Suffice it to say that they are not paid a salary and dispensing of medicines and sales of other goods contribute to their income. From soaps, shampoos and tooth-pastes, most pharmacists have expanded into cosmetics, sun-glasses and health foods; a few have gone further and sell everything from children's clothes to costume jewellery.

Would they be prepared to give up such lucrative trade even if they were offered payment for advising patients about their drugs, carrying out home visits and providing a round-the-clock service, as has been suggested? The gross profit of the average high-street pharmacist who owns his shop is £40,000 but salaries and overheads have to be subtracted from this. An experienced pharmacist who does not own his shop can expect to earn about £15,000 managing someone else's pharmacy. Some pharmacists, those with the larger shops selling the wider ranges of goods, earn far more. It is unlikely that the fees they would earn from new professional duties would compensate for a loss of earnings from other sales.

Some pharmacists have put forward the argument that a greater professional role and the sale of 'fancy goods' need not be mutually exclusive.

Many family doctors boost their incomes by performing extra services for which fees are paid – family planning, immunizations, insurance examinations and so on. They do not lose professional status by making extra money through private practice. So what is wrong with qualified pharmacists advising N H S patients about their drugs in one part of the shop, while unqualified assistants sell children's toys in another part of the store to paying customers?

There are no easy answers, which is why the future role of the retail pharmacist will probably have to evolve over many years and not simply metamorphose overnight. One area where the pharmacist does seem to have carved out a new niche which makes use of his training and provides important complementary skills to those of doctors and nurses has been in hospitals. How has he managed this successful transition and how have patients benefited from his undoubted skills?

Pharmacists in Hospitals

When we go into hospital we tend to get 'taken over'. Meals appear at set times, baths are taken at regular intervals and drugs are handed out with little more explanation than 'it's for your bowels', or 'it'll make you feel better'. Small wonder that anyone who spends more than a few weeks in hospital needs a sort of re-adjustment course when they leave, to enable them to cope unaided with the outside world. Most people will take at least one and often several types of drug with them when they leave hospital. Suddenly, they must know what they are taking, how much to take and how often. And it is the hospital pharmacists who are playing an increasing role in helping patients get to grips with their drugs in readiness for the day they go home.

Some 3700 pharmacists work in hospitals. They order drugs and distribute them to the wards when they are needed. And they make up a wide variety of drugs for patients with specific requirements. Many of these drugs must be used within a few hours of being made and so they cannot come pre-packaged from the drug companies. In addition, many patients in hospital cannot take food by mouth; they need carefully balanced mixtures of nutrients given through a drip in their arm and many of these have to be put together by the hospital pharmacist.

Hospital pharmacists are also an invaluable source of information about drugs for both doctors and nursing staff. Many go on ward rounds with the doctors and advise on medication. They have also been involved in drawing up lists of necessary drugs in hospitals which have their own prescribing policies so that only the most cost-effective medicines are available – rather like the government's limited list. And pharmacists in many of the larger hospitals provide an information service about the drugs available, both to doctors and nursing staff within the hospital and to local GPs and health professionals. They provide information leaflets about groups of drugs, pointing out the advantages and disadvantages of different products, for both hospital and community-based doctors.

Out-patients are frequently prescribed drugs which they can pick up at the pharmacy before leaving the hospital. And pharmacists are on hand to explain the proper use of their drugs to the patients in a streamlined version of the service provided in some chemists' shops.

It has been suggested that the advisory role performed by hospital pharmacists could be extended to other institutions where patients are temporary or permanent residents, such as nursing and old people's homes, psychiatric homes and places caring for the physically or mentally handicapped. Many of these institutions are badly understaffed and stories abound of patients receiving large quantities of tranquillizing drugs to keep them sedated. Yet, with carefully balanced drugs, many patients can lead much fuller lives, even in residential homes, than if they are victims of multiple drugs. Elderly people frequently lose all grip on reality when they enter nursing homes where large amounts of drugs are used. Yet studies have shown that when these drugs are reduced elderly patients can frequently regain many of their faculties previously thought lost for good. Elderly patients, because of their different reactions to drugs, compared with younger people, need their dosages carefully controlled by experts in pharmacology. And many health workers believe that pharmacists, with, inevitably, a greater knowledge of drugs than other medical staff, could have an important role in overseeing drug usage both in residential homes and in the hostels and day-centres to which an increasing number of mentally ill patients are being discharged.

The elderly are making up an ever-increasing proportion of the community, and people skilled in the correct use of drugs for this group are going to be at a premium. Pharmacists are already proving their worth in hospitals and showing they can work alongside doctors, nurses and other health workers to improve drug usage. But the contribution they can make in other residential homes has yet to be fully assessed.

Pharmacists in Health Education

Such has been the antipathy from the medical profession towards the idea of pharmacists taking more responsibility for telling patients about their drugs that pharmacists have taken an even more 'softly, softly' approach to the proposal that they could be involved in other aspects of preventive health care and education.

With the need for pharmacists to make up medicines largely gone why should they not turn their attention to simple diagnostic tests such as checking urine for sugar or performing other laboratory tests, argue the enthusiasts. Screening people for diabetes and keeping an eye on those who have already been diagnosed could easily be done from the pharmacy. The same is true of pregnancy tests and simple blood and urine checks of hormone and other body chemicals. In large American cities almost every shopping precinct has facilities for simple screening procedures for high blood pressure, diabetes, glaucoma, even certain types of cancer. A few years ago, automatic blood-pressure machines were installed in some British pharmacies and department stores amidst uproar from doctors that people would be worried unnecessarily by incorrect high readings or lulled into a false sense of security by inaccurate normal results.

The machines met with a mixed response from the public, most lying idle after the initial novelty wore off. Yet the fact remains that thousands of people with undiagnosed high blood pressure are walking around and possibly running the risk of heart attack or other circulatory problems in later life. If doctors do not have the time or inclination routinely to check their patients for raised blood pressure, could not pharmacists help to do the job?

The same goes for weight problems; approximately one in three people in Britain are over their ideal weight and around 7 per cent of adults sufficiently overweight to endanger their health.

Some GPs run diet clinics and health-and-fitness centres are springing up all over the country. But again, could not pharmacists contribute to the move towards better diet by providing simple advice from their shops? Help in giving up smoking could also come into the overall health package. Also, pharmacists, with their considerable knowledge of contraceptive methods, could advise about the barrier methods sold in their shops and the other methods available only from the doctor or family-planning clinic.

Is this taking the role of the pharmacist too far? Should not health education and preventive care be the responsibility of the doctor, practice nurse and health visitor? Doctors' attitudes to preventive care vary; some hold regular diet clinics, blood-pressure screening sessions, well-women and -baby clinics. But others feel they have barely time to see their patients who are ill let alone those who are apparently glowing with good health.

So there is clearly room for other health professionals to play a part in the overall care of the patient, not just when he is sick. Is the pharmacist the right person to take on part of this work?

His knowledge of the anatomy and physiology of the body puts him in good stead. And the greater emphasis on talking with patients which has been making steady inroads into the teaching of the pharmacy student should put him more at ease with those who come into his shop. There is no doubt that the customer has considerable faith in the pharmacist, even if he is not always aware of the full range of health matters on which the pharmacist is qualified to advise. So, why not the pharmacist?

If the pharmacist is to play a greater role in health care then he will also have to take responsibility when things go wrong. Pharmacists' leaders were secretly rather pleased when a pharmacist was held partly responsible, and had to pay compensation in a recent court case involving a prescription for a drug commonly used for the treatment of migraine. The doctor made an error in the dose written on the prescription and this was not picked up by the pharmacist; the patient suffered gangrene in her feet and had to have some of her toes amputated. The judge decided that both doctor and pharmacist were equally to blame and awarded £100,000 in compensation. The doctor had to pay

£45,000, one of his colleagues had to pay £15,000 and the pharmacist £40,000.

A precedent has therefore been set and pharmacists can expect to be held responsible in future for errors which slip through their hands. If we are to be held responsible in law, argue the pharmacists, we must have a more clearly defined role in the prescribing and dispensing of drugs to the public.

However, before pharmacists take on any new role, they must be seen to be getting their present job right. A recent survey by the Consumers Association revealed a disturbing number of pharmacists handing out poor advice. Either they failed to recommend that patients see their doctor when symptoms merited a visit to the surgery, or they advised patients too freely to buy medicines from the pharmacy when dietary or other advice would have been more appropriate. Be sure that pharmacists are following current guidance before extending their role, was the advice of the Consumers Association.

Not every pharmacist wants to take on a greater role in the care of the patient, even in providing more information about drugs – let alone screening for things like diabetes and high blood pressure. To some extent it is the new, young pharmacists fresh out of university and filled with the latest thinking on the correct use of drugs, who want to take more responsibility for their patients. Many of the older pharmacists are quite content to continue until retirement in their present role. Unlike doctors, there is no incentive for pharmacists to attend postgraduate refresher or training courses once they leave college. But clearly, if the pharmacists are to take a greater role in diagnosing and prescribing for minor illnesses they will need some form of follow-up training.

The plea by pharmacists for a greater role in health care is not new. They have been a profession without a proper job description for fifteen to twenty years. And there are now a substantial proportion of pharmacists who have not had to do more than transfer tablets from one bottle to another, with no need for making up medicines themselves, since they finished their training. But it seems that the much underrated talents of the pharmacist may at last be put to better use and his valuable training properly exploited.

CHAPTER 9

A Matter of Choice

The pharmaceutical industry spends about £180 million each year, promoting its drugs to Britain's doctors. This promotion takes many forms – advertising, leaflets through the letter-box, visits from representatives and sponsorship of events.

Is there anything wrong with this? All industries have a sales force; how else are they to introduce potential buyers to their products and make their sales? The question for the medical profession is whether doctors rely too heavily on promotional literature to find out about the relative merits of new drugs and not enough on other, more rigorous, assessments. Drug companies do have enormous amounts of information about their drugs at their disposal. After all, it was they who did the research and development. But as in any industry, their promotional literature tends to highlight the advantages of their drugs and play down the drawbacks.

In most industries, that is considered fair play; let the buyer beware. But health is different. Playing up effectiveness or playing down side-effects is not acceptable when it is a patient's health and not just a bonus form which is at stake. Should the burden be on the doctor to be sure he asks the right question of his rep or examines the small print of the advertisements? Often there are only subtle differences between drugs or a drug may be so new that little is known of its relative merits. How then can doctors decide? They like to think that they are not influenced by the drug advertisements they see in their medical journals. But you only have to talk to them about some of the most striking advertisements to find that they have taken in more than they thought. Every year drug advertisements win prizes for their imagination and ingenuity – if not their subtlety.

Companies are only allowed to advertise drugs to the public which are bought direct from the chemist. They cannot advertise prescription medicines in ordinary newspapers and magazines and must restrict themselves to journals like the *Lancet* and the *British Medical Journal* which will only be read by those with medical qualifications. But there are other ways of ensuring that we all hear about new drugs, often before our doctors. Journalists are invited to conferences and laboratories and word soon trickles through of the newest drug for arthritis, the latest thing for losing weight or another way of treating cancer. Companies have not been slow to exploit such additional sources of pressure on doctors to prescribe their drugs. Where advertisements and other promotion have failed to influence prescribing, a plea from a chronically sick patient who has read about a new drug may do the trick.

Less than half the pharmaceutical industry's promotional budget is spent on advertisements. Far more is spent on the sales force which preaches direct to the doctor, and on sponsoring medical meetings for doctors and holding conferences. In recent years, it is these latter activities which have come in for the greatest criticism. An all-expenses-paid trip on the Orient Express for a group of rheumatologists was the beano which hit the headlines but dozens of smaller-scale entertainments are staged in desirable overseas locations each year, away from the glare of publicity.

What Are These Events and How Can They Be Justified?

Behind such trips there is usually a new drug which the company wants to promote to the doctors or an ailing drug which the company is trying to revive in the face of fierce competition from newer products. What happens is this. The drug company sponsors a conference about the drug, generally over a weekend and frequently in Europe – Zurich has always been a favourite and so has Milan. But recently companies became so enamoured of Portugal that there was scarcely a room to be had for the tourists in one desirable resort!

Having decided on its location, the company chooses its delegates carefully. Ideally, it wants a mixture of doctors who have used its latest drug already and some whom it wishes to initiate.

That way, the two groups will mix and the well-versed doctors will pass on the good news, and the novices will not feel they have been brainwashed by the drug company. One of the two days of the weekend meeting will be devoted to the conference. The subtler companies will include a couple of papers which do not discuss their new drug directly. If the meeting concerns hypertension, for example, they will begin with a couple of papers on what causes high blood pressure, the treatments already available and what will happen to people whose pressure remains uncontrolled. It will only be after coffee that they move on to the most serious stuff, referring to the new drug. And the post-luncheon presentations will be just extra padding for those keen enough to have stayed on and avoided the lure of the beach or shops.

Frequently, these meetings are held as so-called satellite symposia to major international conferences held under the auspices of academic societies. In return for financial support in holding these expensive meetings, the drug companies are allowed to hold their mini-symposia alongside the major conference. That way, they are able to invite some of their own delegates and they hope to attract other doctors at the meeting who drift from hall to hall at the conference in search of something to interest them. They will also be able to get better speakers than they might otherwise be able to do if they held their conference separately. Leading figures in the relevant area of medicine may be persuaded to speak at the drug-company symposia because they will be at the major meeting anyway, whereas they might be less tempted by a time-consuming meeting at some other location at a different date.

Do Such Meetings Really Influence Prescribing Habits?

It is difficult to quantify how influential these meetings are. No one has ever followed doctors up after they get back from such a trip to see if they immediately start prescribing the drug they have just heard about. But the fact that companies are prepared to go on funding such meetings suggests that they see some benefit. Equally, it could be said that such meetings will only influence a doctor's prescribing if the new drug actually works. She may hand the latest anti-arthritic agent out to the first half-dozen patients who come into her surgery, but if they come back complaining that their arthritis is worse then she will soon stop prescribing it.

Problems arise when the new drug is as good as or even marginally better than similar products, but it is more expensive and proves to have more serious side-effects. Over a million prescriptions for the anti-arthritic drug, Opren, are thought to have been handed out in the relatively short period it was on the market, such was the effectiveness of the company's promotional activities. It has been argued that if the drug had been released more slowly fewer people need have suffered side-effects before the dangers were recognized.

Is promotional material from the drug company – whether in the form of leaflets through the letter-box or international conferences – the right way of introducing doctors to a new drug and informing them fully of both the advantages and the disadvantages? What other sources of information are available?

The DHSS pays for all doctors to be sent a handbook of drugs called the *British National Formulary*. This is put together by experts twice a year and classifies drugs according to their cost and effectiveness. The DHSS also pays for the *Drug and Therapeutics Bulletin* which is produced fortnightly and which gives an in-depth analysis of drugs in specific areas of medicine. Doctors also get, free of charge, the *Prescribers Journal* which consists of series of short articles on areas of current therapeutic interest. The DHSS puts out occasional warnings about drugs and the chief medical officer writes to each doctor when a particularly worrying issue arises or a drug is to be withdrawn from the market. But the rest of the time, the doctor must rely on what he reads in the journals, hears at conferences or is told by drug companies.

This is not to say that doctors spend their free time on an endless round of overseas beanos. There are plenty of doctors who have never accepted more than a coffee and a sandwich from a drug company. But they say you can tell how many 'freebies' a doctor has been on by the depth of his tan.

It is not all as one-sided as it sounds either. There are doctors who are only too keen to work the system; the same faces turn up at every freebie from Paris to Rome, New York to Bangkok. Many is the drug-company executive who has been heard to mutter over the endless capacity of some doctors to enjoy the good life and pass on the expenses to their benefactors. Some believe they have made a rod for their own back; by starting the practice of overseas conferences and other benefits they have encouraged doctors to expect ever higher standards of bonhomie. And now it is too late to stop.

Back home some doctors are only too keen to accept anything put in front of them. Drug-company representatives tell stories of doctors taking left-over food home in 'doggy bags'; of delegates removing anything from exhibitions and demonstrations which is not nailed down; even of one rep having to take a valuable piece of medical equipment to the toilet with her in case it disappeared from her stand at an exhibition while she was out of the room. Tales such as these do little to enhance the reputation of the medical profession or encourage confidence in their judgement. There are rotten apples in every barrel, but certain professions – doctors, lawyers, policemen, the clergy, for example – are supposed to be above reproach. Since no one is totally immune to temptation, what official controls are set on the largesse which drug companies can hand out to doctors?

The drug industry operates under a code of practice drawn up by its umbrella organization, the Association of the British Pharmaceutical Industry. On the question of hospitality it says: 'The level of hospitality should be appropriate and not out of proportion to the occasion; its cost should not exceed that level which the recipients might normally adopt when paying for themselves ...', and it adds: 'Hospitality which becomes little more than pure entertainment has limited value in terms of the provision of information and promotion; such hospitality can only be regarded, therefore, as irrelevant and wasteful.'

The code covers all aspects of conduct of drug companies and their representatives from training to advertising, free samples to market research. Complaints against members who breach the code are heard by a committee made up largely of drug-industry executives and two members of the medical profession. Until the last few years decisions on complaints remained secret, known only by the complainant and the defendant. In an effort to cut down on the number of breaches of the code, the Association decided to make its decisions more public in the hope that this would act as a deterrent to others. The problem is that so many companies do breach the code to a lesser or greater degree that being found guilty is more like joining a hall of fame than being put up for public condemnation.

Most of the complaints come from other member companies and the majority refer to breaches of the code referring to advertisements which would sound petty to the outside observer. At the end of 1983 the DHSS sent out a warning to companies because so many of them were making unsubstantiated claims for their drugs in promotional material that things were getting out of hand. But recent surveys have shown continuing infringements. Rarely do complaints refer to hospitality at overseas conferences; there seems to be an unwritten law between companies not to tell tales. Presumably this is because no one would be above reproach if mafia-style vendettas were started up.

In addition to the code of practice, the DHSS has imposed cash limits on the amount of money which companies can spend on promotional activities. Overall, they are now allowed to spend some nine per cent of their turnover on promotion. This has meant a reduction for most companies, over the last two years. Cutbacks have occurred mainly in the amount spent on advertising direct to doctors in medical journals, and has had much less effect on sponsored meetings and medical representatives.

Can Medicine Do without Drug-company Money?

Doctors do need conferences, both local and international, to help them keep up to date about new methods of diagnosis and treatment and to exchange ideas with their colleagues. The same is true of most professions, but particularly of medicine. Such meetings cost money to organize and it can be expensive for doctors to get to them, particularly the overseas meetings.

Medicine is not alone in having industrial sponsors, and without money from drug companies many meetings of specialist associations would not be possible. Likewise, without drug advertising some medical journals would disappear, the only alternative being to increase subscriptions to an unacceptable level. It could be argued that the disappearance of some of the smaller societies and minor medical journals would be no great loss. How many organizations for cardiologists or magazines for rheumatologists do you need? Indeed, the standard of presentation at meetings of some of the smaller societies and papers in the smaller journals can be so poor that their scientific value is questionable.

Conferences and magazines are not the only areas where drug-company sponsorship can be important. Academic research depends increasingly on money from the pharmaceutical industry. This takes two forms. In a relatively small number of cases, drug companies fund specific research projects on drugs. Most of this type of research, however, can be done by the companies themselves in their own laboratories, frequently with the type of equipment that researchers based in universities can only dream of. Much more drug-company money goes to research departments based in hospitals which do trials of new drugs on patients. Once they have completed laboratory and animal studies on new drugs, companies rely on hospitals to test them on human patients. Drug companies prefer their clinical trials to be done in British hospitals since standards are higher than in many overseas countries and results tend to carry more weight with governments handing out licences for new drugs than if trials are done elsewhere.

Hospital departments are relying increasingly on the money they are paid for such trials to pay for new equipment and even the salaries of researchers. In recent years over 150 academic jobs have been lost because of cuts in government funding. Charities which provide money for research into specific diseases also need money from drug companies to hand on for research.

Just how much money is provided by the industry for drug research in hospitals and universities is unknown. But it has cemented the links between the drug industry and the medical profession and there can be few major academic departments doing drug research which do not rely to a greater or lesser degree on the drug industry.

Medical research needs the drug industry and the drug industry needs the help of British doctors. But unless the two partners can keep their relationship on a totally professional basis they will lose credibility. Some leading academics have already expressed doubts about the role of the drug industry in research and in sponsoring medical conferences and other events, and they fear that patients will lose faith in their doctors if they believe they are being influenced in the drugs they prescribe.

Patients expect to be prescribed what is best for them and they expect their doctor's decision to be based on their illness, the drugs which are available, the risks of side-effects and the doctor's previous experience. They do not expect an advertising campaign, a visit from a persuasive rep or a weekend in Cannes to come into the equation.

How Can We Choose?

Doctors are not the only ones who are bombarded with advertisements about drugs. We cannot open a magazine or switch on the television without being told of the most powerful pain-killer or the most effective cold cure. The products are different from those the doctors are told about but the technique is the same – buy ours, it's better!

The drug industry spends some £50 million a year advertising drugs which can be bought at chemists' shops, supermarkets and other retail outlets. That is 8 per cent of the total market for these so-called over-the-counter drugs, which stands at around £400 million a year.

If doctors find it difficult to weigh up the claims made about drugs, how much harder it is for us to decide which product will do us some good. The Independent Broadcasting Authority (IBA) checks on the standards of advertisements which appear on television, and manufacturers of over-the-counter medicines also have a code of conduct which covers advertising both in newspapers and magazines and on television and radio. In fact, it is much tougher than the code which governs advertising to doctors since manufacturers have to submit their advertisements to their umbrella organization, the Proprietary Association of Great Britain (PAGB), for approval before they can release them. In the case of advertisements to doctors, the Association of the

British Pharmaceutical Industry only responds to complaints about advertisements after they are published.

The PAGB represents manufacturers of about 90 per cent of drugs sold over the counter in the United Kingdom. It is not the only body which keeps a watchful eye over advertising to the public. The Code of Advertising Practice Committee plays a similar role for advertising in magazines and newspapers to that of the IBA for advertising on television. The DHSS also keeps tabs on the claims made by drugs companies in advertisements to the public.

It is curious that while advertising to doctors has taken on a more Sunday-colour-supplement approach in recent years, consumer advertising has become more 'scientific'. While the doctors get concept-oriented advertisements which use animals, trains, fire, water to put across power, strength or tranquillity we get the men in white coats with test tubes who stamp 'proved' across their products. But this is pseudo-science. There are no real comparisons with the effectiveness of other products. Doctors do at least see the results of studies which compare one drug against another in the treatment of any given disease. But we are left to carry out our own comparisons. We try a pain-killer and if it works we stick to it; if it does not we try something else. But for us to have heard about it in the first place means we will probably have seen it advertised, which means it will be one of the leading brands, which in turn means it will probably be one of the more expensive brands. The simplest, and cheapest, brands of most over-the-counter drugs are not advertised.

Manufacturers of over-the-counter drugs are rarely allowed to compare their products with rival medicines, either by suggesting greater effectiveness or by pointing out the presence or absence of specific components of the products. So a manufacturer of a pain-killer containing paracetamol cannot say, in an advertisement, that it does not contain aspirin, and vice versa.

There is considerable debate over whether companies should be allowed to make comparisons in their advertisements. In America, it is a case of no holds barred. Almost every advertisement on television appears to knock someone else's product. But it seems to be a curiously British trait not to compare a product with its rivals in advertising. A few subtle comparisons have begun to creep in but washing-powder and margarine advertisements, for example, still coyly compare the products with 'another leading brand'.

Drug manufacturers are only allowed to compare their products with rivals when they can properly substantiate their claims. And it is felt that we, the consumers, should not be expected to make judgements about the relative merits of medicines based on scientific information in advertisements. Because we do not have the background knowledge it would be impossible to judge who was telling the truth. Yet if the IBA and the Proprietary Association of Great Britain can decide whether the advertising we are currently shown is misleading, could they not make more effort to judge advertising which compares rival products? At least then we would have a better idea of which product was most suitable for us – rather than being bombarded with different claims.

It has been argued that advertisements are meant only as a reminder of a product and that most people decide what drug they are going to buy on the basis of recommendations from their friends, colleagues at work, or pharmacists. And so advertisements are not the proper place for comparisons of products. Yet £50 million seems an awful lot to spend on reminders.

So where else can we get information about the relative merits of different medicines? There are no equivalents for the general public of the *British National Formulary* and the *Drug and Therapeutics Bulletin* which keep doctors informed about current thinking on drugs – their advantages and disadvantages. Magazine and newspaper articles tend to concentrate on miracle breakthroughs or drug disasters.

Limitations put on the drugs which can be prescribed by the doctor on the NHS have only added to the confusion over drugs we can buy from the chemist. A large number of cough and cold remedies, vitamins and tonics which were previously available on prescription and could also be bought from the chemist's shop are now available only from the chemist. Many of these products, previously promoted exclusively to doctors because their over-the-counter market was relatively small, are now finding their way into advertisements in magazines and newspapers. These products were always available to us, we just were not aware of

them. Now, they are fighting for a share of a market previously
sewn up by the big-name brands. And we must try and weigh the
claims of these products against the vast range of medicines
already packing the pharmacy shelves.

What should we be looking for in a simple pain-killer for a
head or stomach ache? What do we need for an upset stomach? Is
it worth buying something for a cold or would we do just as well
with a whisky and hot lemon?

Simple Pain-killers

In 1984 we spent £85 million on pain-killers bought from
chemists', supermarkets and other shops – some £7 million more
than the previous year. The most widely sold pain-killer, so the
advertisements keep telling us, is Anadin. This contains a mixture
of aspirin, caffeine and quinine. Is it really any more effective in
relieving pain than a simple aspirin, costing less than a third of
the price?

Pharmacologists are regularly baffled by studies which show
that branded pain-killers with a mixture of ingredients are more
effective than simple aspirin or paracetamol. In most cases, there
is no scientific reason why there should be any additional benefit
and the difference has to be attributed to the expectations of
patients. We all have an in-built feeling that if it costs more it
must be better. And while we may be prepared to sacrifice quality
in furniture, clothing, hi-fi equipment, even food, when it comes
to medicine we want the best – and we are prepared to pay for it.
But are we really buying better?

The difference between pain-killers is more of packaging than
content. Most pain-killers contain either aspirin, paracetamol or
codeine. Many people now prefer to take paracetamol rather
than aspirin because it is less likely to cause stomach irritation
and indigestion. People seem to believe that codeine is reserved
for more severe pain but it is sold in much smaller doses than
those used by doctors to treat chronic pain, when there is a small
risk of addiction from the drug.

There is a definite move towards the use of soluble rather than
insoluble versions of pain-killers because of their reduced risk of
stomach problems. And here, some of the branded products may

have advantages in appearance, if not in effect. They dissolve totally in water to give a completely clear solution rather than leaving a milky-looking liquid, with bits of undissolved drug floating in it. Many people, particularly children, prefer the clear, tasteless solution to the cloudier liquid (which frequently has some taste to it as well), even if it costs considerably more.

Other formulations also have their fans. Some people find tablets hard to swallow and prefer capsules which slip down more easily. Others like the convenience of a product which dissolves in the mouth. Syrup formulations of pain-killers for children may not do wonders for their teeth but at least they help children take the drugs. The same is true of pain-killers which can be chewed. Some pain-killers have stimulants such as caffeine added but frequently in such small amounts that they would have less effect than a cup of coffee.

And other products contain two types of pain-killer – aspirin and paracetamol or paracetamol and codeine. So are they twice as effective? That rather depends on the amount of each drug in the product and the recommended dose. If you actually take the trouble to take half the pain-killers in the shop off the shelves and compare how much of each component is in each product you will often find that where drugs are combined the amount of each component in the product is less than if it was sold on its own, or the dose is lower or less frequent.

In general, doctors do not like these so called 'combination' drugs, because they cannot be sure how the components will interact with each other once they are in the body and how much of each one will be released. They prefer to increase the dose of a single pain-killer up to the recommended dose rather than to start using combinations of drugs. If you are in such severe pain that a simple aspirin or paracetamol preparation, taken at the maximum recommended dose, is not working then you should see your doctor and not try taking combinations of pain-killers.

Certain types of pain do respond better to one pain-killer rather than another. When the anti-inflammatory drug, ibuprofen, recently became available from chemists', as well as on prescription, people with muscular pain were able to buy a particularly effective drug for such problems, without having to go to the doctor. Advertisements announcing the drug as a breakthrough in pain relief did seem rather outdated as the drug has been available on prescription for many years. However, that is not to detract from the drug's effectiveness. But people with chronic arthritis whose prescribed drugs are not entirely effective should be aware that at some time they will almost certainly have been prescribed ibuprofen or a very similar drug by their doctor. And if it did not work then, it probably will not work now. So they should not be too optimistic even if the advertisements do call it a breakthrough. Ibuprofen is also very useful for the treatment of period pain. Again, doctors have been prescribing anti-inflammatory drugs such as ibuprofen for some years to women whose period pain is not controlled by aspirin or other simple pain-killers. It does not work for everyone but it can be highly effective.

Cough and Cold Remedies

Aspirin and paracetamol form the mainstay of the majority of cold remedies. Even the most optimistic of manufacturers has given up suggesting that its products actually cure colds and flu; the emphasis now is on relief of symptoms. It is a line which works, since second only to pain-killers we spend more on cough and cold remedies than any other drugs bought from chemists – around £65 million worth in 1984.

The pain-killers, in addition to relieving aching limbs in colds and flu, also lower temperature and reduce fever. Since it is often the raised temperature, more than anything else, which makes us feel ill with a cold or flu, products containing aspirin, paracetamol or codeine all have their place in simple self-medication. As with analgesics, the simple remedies containing single drugs are preferred by doctors.

Many cold remedies also contain a nasal decongestant, most commonly phenylephrine or phenylpropanolamine. Both these drugs have come in for considerable criticism because they raise blood pressure. They should not be taken by anyone with hypertension or diabetes or people taking certain types of anti-depressant drugs.

Pseudoephedrine is another drug which has come under close scrutiny in the last few years because of reports that it can cause hallucinations in young children. A report in one of the medical journals of children who hallucinated about snakes and spiders triggered a series of similar reports. Pseudoephedrine is related to ephedrine which has been used by drug abusers for its hallucinogenic properties. Pseudoephedrine is found in a number of common cough mixtures, the best known being Actifed. And although the hallucinations appear to be relatively rare, parents should be aware that these can occur if they are planning to give the drug to young children. Alternatively, they may prefer to choose something which does not contain the drug.

If you are planning to buy a cough mixture decide whether you want something to soothe or to encourage coughing. Some products contain both a cough suppressant and an expectorant – something which encourages coughing – and such combinations do appear to defy all reasonable logic. Most coughs go away of their own accord within a week or so of a cold, so there may be no need for a cough mixture. But if you do decide to buy a cough medicine, something to soothe a cough should contain either noscapine, dextromethorphan or pholcodine while an expectorant will probably contain sodium citrate or terpin hydrate.

A sore throat is often one of the worst aspects of having a cold and many of the pastilles and lozenges on the market taste so nice that people do not wait for a bad throat to buy them. Since it is relief from pain you are after, aspirin or paracetamol should do the job just as well, or honey and hot lemon for a soothing combination. The latest thing for colds, which is claimed to reduce their duration, if not actually cure them, is zinc. Even the experts at Britain's Common Cold Unit think there may be something in this particular remedy but they are waiting for more evidence before they come down totally in its favour. You do not have to chew on a lump of metal to poison the virus, you can buy the zinc in tablet form. The difficult thing may be to prove that the zinc really does reduce the length of a cold. People vary in how long they feel ill. But most people feel better within a week, so any 'cure' must show that it can reduce the cold by several days, otherwise it probably is not worth using.

Vitamins

Love them or hate them, vitamins account for around £30 million worth of over-the-counter drug sales each year, and that does not include vitamins bought at health-food stores. There can be few areas of medicine which excite such passion as vitamins; the majority of the medical profession see them as a waste of money for all but a tiny minority of people with deficiencies, while the new breed of health fanatic swears by them. A recent survey showed that the biggest consumers of vitamins are female, middle class and in the healthiest of age groups, 16–34. Just the group, says medical opinion, least likely to be vitamin deficient. Young children, the elderly and certain ethnic groups are the only people thought not to get sufficient vitamins from their normal diet.

Around 5 per cent of Britons take vitamins regularly, though as many as one in four people are thought to take them from time to time. Even this is nothing compared to the 40 per cent of Americans who take them regularly. Multivitamins are the most popular, though a recent edition of the *Drug and Therapeutics Bulletin* recommended that people buy cheaper single vitamins if they had to buy vitamins at all. But most experts stand by the view that, provided all the vitamins are not cooked out of food by prolonged boiling, all our requirements can be found in an average diet.

Vitamin A is found in green vegetables, carrots, liver and dairy products and is needed for healthy skin, hair and nails. B vitamins are found in raw vegetables, milk, eggs, fruit and yeast and are important for good mental health since a deficiency can lead to depression, insomnia and lethargy. Vitamin C is found in large quantities in fresh fruit and was first identified in preventing scurvy. Vitamin D is found in fish, liver and milk and is needed for healthy teeth and bones and, finally, vitamin E is present in some vegetable oils and green vegetables and has fabled youth-giving properties.

The B and C vitamins are probably most frequently taken as supplements in spite of the fact that the body has little capacity for storing more than its immediate requirements for them and excretes any excess in urine. This is particularly true of vitamin C but large numbers of people remain convinced that they can prevent colds with large quantities of the vitamin. In spite of the support for this theory from Nobel prize-winner, Linus Pauling, there is little real evidence in favour of it.

There are B vitamins for sale which have never even been scientifically recognized. In fact a vitamin should, by definition, be essential to nutrition which many of the so-called B vitamins certainly are not. In fact, vitamin B17, which is still used in some controversial cancer clinics, is known to be toxic. And doubts hang over some of the other more obscure B group.

Vitamin B6 has taken on a new lease of life with the discovery that it can relieve symptoms of premenstrual tension. Vitamin E has also found favour in medical circles for helping to prevent blindness in very premature babies and possibly even in preventing brain haemorrhages in these children. But these are highly specialized uses – a far cry from using it to avoid wrinkles. Again, medical experts are highly sceptical about how a vitamin slapped on the skin can penetrate the surface and bring new life to old cells. Vitamin A taken in large doses is dangerous.

Pregnant women are now given multiple vitamins since it was shown that they could prevent the birth of babies with spina bifida. Further research is being carried out to confirm the earlier findings and you should be advised by your doctor about which vitamins to take. Another small group who do need vitamins are Asian women and children who eat a vegetarian diet and rarely expose their skin to sunlight. They are frequently deficient in vitamin D, which is activated by sunlight, and need supplements in order to avoid bone deformities such as rickets. Strict vegetarians may also need some additional vitamin supplements since they will miss out on vitamins in meat, fish and dairy products. But again, anyone with a vitamin deficiency caused by their diet should be seeing a doctor to ensure that they get the vitamins right, not dosing themselves on vitamins bought at the chemist.

There is little doubt that people do take vitamins unnecessarily but, equally, they are probably so convinced that they are doing them good that they do actually feel better. Another victory for the powers of the mind over medicine!

Laxatives

One of the few categories of drugs where over-the-counter sales are flattening off, if not actually dropping, are laxatives. Sales have held steady at around the £10 million mark for the last few years. The optimists amongst the medical profession are attributing the trend to better eating habits. Perhaps the message about eating plenty of high-fibre food is getting through.

Over the years, constipation has become something of a national institution. And there are plenty of people around who were given liquid paraffin or syrup of figs on a Friday night to keep them regular. In fact it kept most of them in the toilet – and out of trouble – for most of Saturday morning.

There are four main types of drug for constipation. First there are so-called 'bulking agents' such as products containing methyl cellulose or ispaghula granules which, as the name implies, help in the formation of stools. The extra stools then stimulate the bowel into action. They tend to take longer to relieve constipation than some drugs and they can give a feeling of 'fullness' in the abdomen and wind. Second there are drugs which will soften the stools and make them easier to pass. Such products include drugs such as liquid paraffin and docusate sodium. These are especially useful to help patients with constipation and piles.

The third group of drugs for constipation are those which stimulate the bowel to move directly. Senna is probably the best known example of this group of drugs. Many people, particularly the elderly and those who do not get much exercise, have a slow-moving bowel and drugs may be needed to stir it into action. But these drugs are best avoided by young children and pregnant women. The final group are called osmotic laxatives. These have the advantage of being fast-acting but they are frequently abused by dieters trying to lose weight. The most well-known of this group of drug are lactulose and magnesium salts.

Laxatives should never be seen as an alternative to a good diet with plenty of fruit, vegetables and cereals and sufficient exercise to keep the bowel awake. Drugs very quickly become a routine and so it is preferable to put a little bran on breakfast cereal or to eat cereals already containing extra bran. Most food manufacturers have become adept at masking the taste of bran on its own. If simple dietary measures are not effective then short courses of laxatives can work very well. If constipation persists, however, you should consult a doctor to check that there is no underlying disease requiring treatment.

Medicines for Indigestion

We may be eating more fibre and managing to avoid constipation but we are still eating the fatty foods which give us indigestion – to the tune of £26 million worth of drugs each year. Most of us get by with a simple antacid to counteract the excessive acid secretion in the stomach. But some people go on to develop ulcers which require medicines only available on prescription.

There are dozens of indigestion remedies on the market and, as with pain-killers and cough and cold remedies, the cheaper, simpler drugs are probably just as effective as the more expensive products which contain a variety of drugs. Most of these antacids contain either aluminium hydroxide, or salts of magnesium or sodium; in fact, bicarbonate of soda must be in virtually everyone's kitchen or medicine cabinet.

The aluminium and magnesium salts are slower-acting but go on working for longer than sodium salts. The sodium salts also have the disadvantage that they cannot be given to people on low-sodium diets such as those with kidney or heart problems. The aluminium-based drugs tend to cause constipation and the magnesium salts diarrhoea. None of them should be taken with other medicines as they may impair their absorption or interact with them. Formulations of these products vary and people may base their preference on the ease with which the drugs can be used, and chewy products are popular for this reason.

As with constipation, regular, painful indigestion accompanied by regurgitation of acids in the stomach should not be ignored. If there is an ulcer it may require more effective drugs and ulcers can only be confirmed through proper investigation by a doctor.

Diarrhoea and Vomiting

The best treatment for a bout of diarrhoea and vomiting lasting two or three days is no food and plenty of fluids. Drugs bought from the chemist frequently serve only to prolong the infection in the long term because they stop the removal of the offending organism from the body. A stomach upset continuing for more than a few days may require a visit from the doctor particularly if there is vomiting as well as diarrhoea, because people can quickly become very dehydrated. This is why it is so important to drink plenty of fluids to replace the water lost.

Diarrhoea and vomiting in babies, people with chronic illnesses and the elderly also need special attention and a visit from the doctor, as all these groups can go downhill quickly when they become severely dehydrated.

'Don't eat and take plenty of fluids' may seem like good advice; it may also be totally impractical. If you are travelling by train across Egypt with all the toilet facilities for which such countries are renowned you probably will not be able simply to let the infection take its course. The most commonly used and effective drugs for these circumstances are kaolin and morphine, taken separately or together. Kaolin has the effect of making the loose fecal material bind together and morphine slows down the movement of the gut. Neither drug gets rid of the bacteria or other organisms causing the infection; it is left to the body's defences either to overpower or expel the organisms. Even when drugs are taken to control diarrhoea, you should not forget to take plenty of liquids and, if possible, avoid solid foods until the upset has settled down.

The number of cases of food poisoning has risen dramatically in Britain in the last few years and this has been blamed on poor kitchen hygiene. It is very important to bring all meat to boiling point during cooking, whether during roasting or reheating. Cooked meat should never be stored in the fridge alongside uncooked meat as the bacteria may be transferred to the cooked meat and consumed if the meat is eaten cold. Pork, chicken and shellfish are common places for bacteria to be found; and even using the same utensils for cutting or chopping cooked and uncooked meat, without thorough washing in between, is asking for trouble. Food poisoning is yet another example of prevention being better than cure.

Drugs for Acne

There can be few people who pass through adolescence without at some time venturing into the chemists' for something for their spots. Those with the most severe acne will need drugs that are only available on prescription – and even then they may not be successful.

But for the simpler skin problems a combination of cleansing solutions and products to unblock pores is probably sufficient. Most products contain benzoyl peroxide, salicylic acid, sulphur or chlorhexidine. It is important to keep the skin clean so that there is less chance of pores becoming blocked and encouraging organisms to grow and set up the vicious circle of spot formation, healing and re-forming. Many people find that avoiding certain foods such as fatty products and chocolate can help reduce the risk of spots. It does not help to be told you will grow out of it and many prescription medicines are very effective. But some people do have to wait until they are through the acne age group.

Summary

The list above is not meant to be comprehensive but it does give some idea of the kind of medicines which doctors think are worth buying if we are looking for symptomatic relief of minor illnesses. At the end of the day it is left to us to choose which medicine we think will do us most good. We may remain convinced that a well-known branded pain-killer is more effective than a cheaper generic equivalent. Or that an expensive cough mixture really does get rid of our cough.

The choice is ours. But at least we should be aware of what is available and the fact that 'cheap' does not necessarily mean substandard or that 'expensive' means better.

CHAPTER 10

The Need for Change

A new poster started appearing in GPs' surgeries in 1985 advising women to tell their doctor if they were pregnant or trying to have a baby. The posters were the culmination of a two-year campaign by members of the Crosby Women's Action Group to prevent pregnant women from being given drugs which could harm their unborn baby. Why were they so determined? One of their members had recently had a much-wanted baby aborted because of the risk that it might be deformed after she unwittingly took a six-week course of antibiotics for a pelvic infection.

The case sums up two of the recurring themes in this book – the poor communication between doctor and patient about drugs and the false assumption which we all tend to make, that medicines are safe. Drugs may be life-saving, they may improve the quality of life, or they may be a waste of money, but they are never without risk. The government could introduce so many safety tests for new drugs that 90 per cent failed. But the remaining 10 per cent would still have unwanted effects and possibly be dangerous to certain groups of people.

The only good thing to come out of the Crosby case was that it showed that a small group of consumers, with no particular knowledge of medicine, could get their views as far as the World Health Organization and push the Health Education Council to produce a poster which might help prevent more women going through the emotional agony of a deformed baby or an unwanted abortion because of the drugs they took in pregnancy.

It should not be so hard for us to get the information we need to take medicines safely. The fault does not lie solely with the doctor either. It is as if we hand over responsibility for our health the moment we go through the surgery door. We manage to negotiate the other hazards of daily life quite effectively but when it comes to drugs we just switch off. Either we assume that we simply would not understand or we take the easy option and pass the buck over to our doctor. In the past, the doctor has accepted the 'guru' role we have given her, and she has been only too happy for us not to question her judgement. But the newer breed of doctor gets much more training in 'communication skills' and is more inclined to put them to the test. She does not want to make all our decisions for us; she wants us to consider some of the options too.

The relationship between doctor and patient is a very important one with an implicit feeling of trust towards the doctor. We know that we can speak freely and in confidence to our doctor and we do not expect details of our consultation to be all over town before we have had time to get out of the surgery. Doctors guard this confidentiality jealously. It is probably even more precious to them than their freedom to prescribe whatever drugs they see fit. The feeling of outrage amongst many family doctors over the Gillick ruling concerning the prescription of contraceptive pills to those under 16 years old showed with what importance doctors regard the principle of confidentiality even in relation to their younger patients.

We also need to feel confident in the drugs we are prescribed. We must know that the doctor has done her homework, that she is up to date with current thinking on the best treatment for our illness, and that she has not been unduly influenced by an advertisement she has seen, a rep she has talked to, or a promotional conference she has attended.

Our doctor should not feel threatened if we ask questions about our treatment, or get her to justify what she has prescribed. Our confidence in our GP will only be undermined if we are not satisfied with our treatment. Our trust is much more likely to be broken if we suffer unexpected side-effects from our drugs than if our doctor admits she is unsure what is wrong with us. On the other hand, if she kept reaching for medical textbooks during our consultation we would become rather worried! But there are limitations on any doctor's diagnostic skills when she is presented with an array of apparently totally unrelated symptoms.

For most of us, learning about biology ended in the fifth year at school and probably got about as far as drawing the insides of a flower and learning how rabbits mate. But there is a growing body of opinion that a little basic education about medicines at school would not go amiss. We learn about the Crusades and the Civil War, sugar-cane production in South America – things that will never touch our daily lives. But we have no idea how an aspirin works or how an antibiotic beats a bacterium. What we know about drug doses we learn from the labels on our medicine bottles – if we are lucky. And what we remember about drug side-effects probably comes from the tragic cases we read about in the newspapers.

Armed with a little basic knowledge of how the body reacts to drugs, we should be able to understand the answers to our questions about our illness; what is wrong, what the drug aims to do, how to take it, and what are the main side-effects. Nor should we be treated like children, being spared knowledge of the risks of the medicines we take. We do not need to be scared witless but we can surely have the advantages and disadvantages of our treatment explained to us.

We would not accept a survey on a house which simply said 'needs a new roof' or an estimate on our car which said 'get a new engine'. We would want to know why the house needed a new roof, whether it could last another few years, how much it would cost. Why should medicines be any different?

There is little doubt that we have been wasting one important source of information – the pharmacist. If our doctor is too busy to explain how to use our drugs, or we forget what she has told us, the pharmacist is in an ideal position to reinforce that information about how to take our medicines. Developments in the way drugs are formulated have added to the pitfalls. Long-acting tablets which release their contents slowly into the body are a boon to those who do not want to have to remember to take them three times a day. But how many people who have difficulty swallowing tablets have been tempted to crush these drugs to help them go down more easily? The effects of such a mistake can be frightening.

For example, a woman crushed a slow-release tablet of a commonly used anti-asthma drug to give to her young brother who did not like swallowing tablets. In normal doses this drug can cause a slight increase in heart rate. Imagine her consternation when the boy's pulse rate hit 200 after taking the drug. In taking the crushed tablet, he had consumed all at once a quantity of drug designed to be released slowly over eight hours – he had swallowed four times the normal dose. The slight increase in heartbeat which might have been expected turned into a frightening gallop and took some time to subside.

It is very easy to make mistakes in the way we take our drugs. We can do things which are so obviously foolish to a doctor that she cannot imagine our doing them, and does not therefore warn us against them. A pharmacist, whose training is geared specifically towards the correct use of drugs and is perhaps more aware of the mistakes we can make in taking our drugs, is in a better position to give us those last warnings and ensure that we know how to take our medicine correctly. We can still get it wrong at home but at least we understood what we should do when we collected our medicine. The pharmacist is also a good 'clearing house' for queries about drugs between visits to the doctor. Often, we do not want to go bothering our doctor with a minor query about the medicine we have been prescribed. And the pharmacist is well equipped to answer those problems. It looks as though the pharmacist will play a much bigger role in advising us about our drugs and, considering the cost of his training and the depths of his knowledge, this is a development to be welcomed.

Drugs may not be the only option open to us. It is true that for those with, say, a severe chest infection, they may be life-saving, and for millions of people with chronic diseases such as hypertension, arthritis or asthma they may mean the difference between being a virtual invalid, scarcely able to move about the house and being able to lead a virtually normal life. But, as we have already seen, there are many conditions where drugs have less to offer. Either they have little effect on the disease itself or their side-effects make them too unpleasant to take. The benefits of the medicine start to be outweighed by the risks. In some cases we can help shift the balance back in our favour by taking precautions. Regular blood-pressure checks and smears for women on the Pill can reduce the risk of circulatory diseases or cervical cancer, just as frequent blood tests for people taking drugs which affect the bone marrow are a safeguard against their running into danger.

Sometimes there is no way of shifting the balance in our favour and then we must think of some alternative. Tranquillizers and sleeping pills may be a useful short-term treatment for acute anxiety or insomnia, but in the longer term the risks of addiction outweigh the likelihood of relief from anxiety or sleeplessness. The alternatives may not suit everyone, but advice and support, counselling, relaxation and psychotherapy are all very real options. Not every doctor offers such services, or access to them through her practice. Many doctors still claim that they do not have time to spend hours with a patient who has emotional problems. But this attitude is passing. Younger doctors, and many of the older ones who have recognized the dangers of tranquillizers, do find time to offer counselling to their patients.

More broadminded doctors will also consider alternative therapies such as osteopathy, acupuncture and homeopathy for their patients. In fact, practitioners of these therapies are tired of being seen as 'alternative'. Not so long ago they were even classified as 'fringe'! They would like their techniques to be complementary to those offered by orthodox medicine. They are still criticized for being unscientific in their methods and failing to do sufficient research to prove that their techniques actually work. Just as charlatans of the nineteenth and early twentieth centuries gave the medical profession a bad name, similarly many 'alternative' therapists have damaged the reputation of osteopaths, acupuncturists and homeopaths.

Homeopathy remains the most difficult of the three major therapies for the medical profession to come to terms with, since it flies in the face of everything that orthodox drugs stand for. Homeopaths fight like with like. They are much more interested in the individual patient's reactions to his disease than the disease itself. While doctors use drugs to influence the body's organs and tissues, the homeopath makes up his remedy to mimic the symptoms experienced by the patient. If the patient is suffering from a headache he will find some natural substance which in toxic amounts is capable of causing a headache. He generally uses the remedy in the tiniest of doses, way below those which would cause the toxic effect and, according to orthodox medicine, way below the amount to have any effect. Often the remedies are so dilute that it is hard to believe there is anything left of the active ingredient. Homeopaths argue that they are not the only ones to fight like with like. Vaccines, for example, use small quantities of an infecting organism to stimulate immune reactions in an individual and hence protect him from later infection. But in spite of enjoying the favour of the Royal Family, homeopathy remains in the realms of magic and witch doctors to most of the medical profession.

Many alternative therapists – including homeopaths – are beginning to put their methods to scientific test. But they also point out that the medical profession has not always been as rigorous in testing its methods as it now requires of the alternative therapists. A large number of medical techniques have simply 'grown up' over the years without ever being put to proper scientific tests. Doctors slowly became aware that one method was better than another and frequently only carried out the clinical trials to prove it long after a technique had come into common usage. Until the introduction of the 1968 Medicines Act there was no requirement for drug companies to prove that their compounds worked or that they were safe.

Just because medicine was less scientifically rigorous in its research in the past is no reason for other therapies not to prove their worth. Doctors are very concerned about patients who turn to alternative therapies to treat serious illnesses which respond to modern medicines; cancer patients, for example, whose tumours are easily treated or cured by drugs who prefer instead to try alternative and unproven remedies. It is very easy, with hindsight, to say 'if only he'd stuck to proper drugs' but many patients do find the thought of some cancer treatments worse than the disease. They would rather take their chance with the alternative therapists whose treatments, they hope, will not have debilitating side-effects than accept what orthodox medicine has to offer. It is crucial, therefore, for us to make such decisions with a full understanding of the facts.

Anti-cancer drugs generally cost more than any other form of medicine. Yet, quite rightly, there is no thought of cost when they are prescribed. No expense should be spared in the treatment of life-threatening diseases. But the same cannot be said for drugs used to treat minor illnesses.

Few of us – doctors included – are aware of how much different medicines cost, or how many drugs are wasted. Courses of treatment tend to be prescribed in the form of thirty or fifty tablets, rarely less. The doctor who prescribes them often fails to consider that the patient might feel better after a week and stop taking them, or that the drugs might not suit him and he will have to come back for something else. The patient too might feel short-changed if he only found half-a-dozen tablets in his medicine bottle after he had paid his standard £2 prescription charge. Yet, each time hospitals ask for old medicines to be returned, they are inundated with thousands of tablets, gallons of medicines, dozens of bottles. It has been estimated that between 5 and 6 per cent of all medicines prescribed in general practice are wasted.

But unused medicines are just one small part of the over-prescribing problem in Britain. A much greater source of waste lies in the number of unnecessary prescriptions handed out each year. Why subject our bodies to chemicals if they do not need them? We are all becoming increasingly aware of what is in our food and the amount of preservatives and additives which have been put in them and we try to buy 'natural' foods instead. Yet tucked in with the weekly shopping are the vitamins to stave off colds, the cough and cold remedies for when the vitamins do not work and the prescription for antibiotics in case the cold turns nasty!

The fault is not ours alone. We blame our doctor for writing the unnecessary prescriptions, our doctor blames us for pressing her into reaching for the prescription-pad. Added to the pressure from us is the doctor's feeling that maybe it is better to be safe than sorry and the fact that she has just read about a new drug which seems to fit the bill nicely. Yet if we knew a little more about the purpose of drugs and our doctors took time to explain that a drug was not needed, would we not all be better off?

The official statistic for people who die while taking normal doses of medicines is a very small number. But no one knows just how many deaths are attributed to other illnesses, where medicines have made a significant contribution. One drug interacting with another, a drug which exacerbates the patient's illness or a drug which triggers some previously dormant disease. Surely it makes sense to reduce such risks by reducing unnecessary exposure to all drugs.

There is also a pounds-and-pence price to pay for our drugs; at £1.6 billion and rising, the government thought it was too high. Whether the restricted list makes the forecast £75 million saving remains to be seen, as does the effect on the health of the drug industry of the cuts in profits imposed by the government. An industry which contributes a trade surplus of nearly £700 million to the balance of payments would normally be seen as a national asset rather than a wicked bogeyman. In fact British drug companies regularly win Queen's Awards for Industry. Making money out of illness does not always leave a bad taste in the mouth. Manufacturers of hospital beds and surgical instruments do not come in for anything like the same criticism as the drug industry. Yet they too are making money out of our misfortunes. They may not make quite the profits made by drug companies but it is not for want of trying!

We do need new and better drugs, but we need them to treat illnesses where at present there are big gaps in treatment. We do not need just more of the same. We need more basic academic research for the many areas of medicine where little is known. Without basic research, drug companies cannot develop the breakthrough drugs. And without the profits from earlier drugs and from less innovative products the industry cannot support the work on new drugs.

If it were just goodies and baddies – we the luckless consumers, they the wicked drug barons – the solutions would be simpler. As it is, safer, more cost-effective use of drugs is something in which we should all play a part – patients, doctors and drug industry.

Useful Addresses

Association of Community Health
  Councils,
Mark Lemon Suite,
Barclays Bank Chambers,
254 Seven Sisters Road,
London N4 2HZ

Consumers Association,
14 Buckingham Street,
London WC2N 6DS

Patients Association,
Room 33,
18 Charing Cross Road,
London WC2H 0HR

College of Health,
18 Victoria Park Square,
Bethnal Green,
London E2 9PF

National Consumer Council,
18 Queen Anne's Gate,
London SW1H 9AA

Tranx,
17 Peel Road,
Harrow,
Middlesex

British Association for Counselling,
37a Sheep Street,
Rugby,
Warwickshire CV21 3BX

Institute for Complementary
  Medicine,
21 Portland Place,
London W1N 3AF

National Marriage Guidance
  Council,
Herbert Gray College,
Little Church Street,
Rugby,
Warwickshire CV21 3AP

The Stress Syndrome Foundation,
Cedar House,
Yalding,
Kent ME18 6JD

Health Rights,
157 Waterloo Road,
London SE1 8XF

Association of Parents of Vaccine
  Damaged Children,
2 Church Street,
Shipston on Stour,
Warwickshire CV36 4AP

Opren Action Group,
13 Carlton Close,
Dereham,
Norfolk NR19 1BS

DHSS,
Alexander Fleming House,
Elephant and Castle,
London SE1 6BY

British Medical Association,
BMA House,
Tavistock Square,
London WC1H 9JP

Association of the British
   Pharmaceutical Industry,
12 Whitehall,
London SW1

Proprietary Association of
   Great Britain,
Vernon House,
Sicilian Avenue,
London WC1

Pharmaceutical Society,
1 Lambeth High Street,
London SE1 7JN

National Pharmaceutical Association,
40–42 St Peter's Street,
St Albans,
Herts

Women's Health Concern,
Ground Floor Flat,
17 Earls Terrace,
London W8 6LP

Index

MORE ABOUT PENGUINS, PELICANS, PEREGRINES AND PUFFINS

For further information about books available from Penguins please write to Dept EP, Penguin Books Ltd, Harmondsworth, Middlesex UB8 0DA.

In the U.S.A.: For a complete list of books available from Penguins in the United States write to Dept DG, Penguin Books, 299 Murray Hill Parkway, East Rutherford, New Jersey 07073.

In Canada: For a complete list of books available from Penguins in Canada write to Penguin Books Canada Ltd, 2801 John Street, Markham, Ontario L3R 1B4.

In Australia: For a complete list of books available from Penguins in Australia write to the Marketing Department, Penguin Books Australia Ltd, P.O. Box 257, Ringwood, Victoria 3134.

In New Zealand: For a complete list of books available from Penguins in New Zealand write to the Marketing Department, Penguin Books (N.Z.) Ltd, Private Bag, Takapuna, Auckland 9.

In India: For a complete list of books available from Penguins in India write to Penguin Overseas Ltd, 706 Eros Apartments, 56 Nehru Place, New Delhi 110019.

PENGUIN REFERENCE BOOKS

☐ *The Penguin Dictionary of Troublesome Words* £2.50

A witty, straightforward guide to the pitfalls and hotly disputed issues in standard written English, illustrated with examples and including a glossary of grammatical terms and an appendix on punctuation.

☐ *The Penguin Guide to the Law* £8.95

This acclaimed reference book is designed for everyday use, and forms the most comprehensive handbook ever published on the law as it affects the individual.

☐ *The Penguin Dictionary of Religions* £4.95

The rites, beliefs, gods and holy books of all the major religions throughout the world are covered in this book, which is illustrated with charts, maps and line drawings.

☐ *The Penguin Medical Encyclopedia* £4.95

Covers the body and mind in sickness and in health, including drugs, surgery, history, institutions, medical vocabulary and many other aspects. Second Edition. 'Highly commendable' – *Journal of the Institute of Health Education*

☐ *The Penguin Dictionary of Physical Geography* £4.95

This book discusses all the main terms used, in over 5,000 entries illustrated with diagrams and meticulously cross-referenced.

☐ *Roget's Thesaurus* £3.50

Specially adapted for Penguins, Sue Lloyd's acclaimed new version of Roget's original will help you find the right words for your purposes. 'As normal a part of an intelligent household's library as the Bible, Shakespeare or a dictionary' – *Daily Telegraph*

A CHOICE OF PENGUINS

☐ *Man and the Natural World* **Keith Thomas** £4.95

Changing attitudes in England, 1500–1800. 'An encyclopedic study of man's relationship to animals and plants . . . a book to read again and again' – Paul Theroux, *Sunday Times* Books of the Year

☐ *Jean Rhys: Letters 1931–66*
 Edited by Francis Wyndham and Diana Melly £4.95

'Eloquent and invaluable . . . her life emerges, and with it a portrait of an unexpectedly indomitable figure' – Marina Warner in the *Sunday Times*

☐ *The French Revolution* **Christopher Hibbert** £4.95

'One of the best accounts of the Revolution that I know . . . Mr Hibbert is outstanding' – J. H. Plumb in the *Sunday Telegraph*

☐ *Isak Dinesen* **Judith Thurman** £4.95

The acclaimed life of Karen Blixen, 'beautiful bride, disappointed wife, radiant lover, bereft and widowed woman, writer, sibyl, Scheherazade, child of Lucifer, Baroness; always a unique human being . . . an assiduously researched and finely narrated biography' – *Books & Bookmen*

☐ *The Amateur Naturalist*
 Gerald Durrell with Lee Durrell £4.95

'Delight . . . on every page . . . packed with authoritative writing, learning without pomposity . . . it represents a real bargain' – *The Times Educational Supplement*. 'What treats are in store for the average British household' – *Daily Express*

☐ *When the Wind Blows* **Raymond Briggs** £2.95

'A visual parable against nuclear war: all the more chilling for being in the form of a strip cartoon' – *Sunday Times*. 'The most eloquent anti-Bomb statement you are likely to read' – *Daily Mail*

A CHOICE OF PENGUINS

☐ *The Complete Penguin Stereo Record and Cassette Guide*
Greenfield, Layton and March   £7.95

A new edition, now including information on compact discs. 'One of the few indispensables on the record collector's bookshelf' – *Gramophone*

☐ *Selected Letters of Malcolm Lowry*
Edited by Harvey Breit and Margerie Bonner Lowry £5.95

'Lowry emerges from these letters not only as an extremely interesting man, but also a lovable one' – Philip Toynbee

☐ *The First Day on the Somme*
Martin Middlebrook   £3.95

1 July 1916 was the blackest day of slaughter in the history of the British Army. 'The soldiers receive the best service a historian can provide: their story told in their own words' – *Guardian*

☐ *A Better Class of Person* **John Osborne**   £2.50

The playwright's autobiography, 1929–56. 'Splendidly enjoyable' – John Mortimer. 'One of the best, richest and most bitterly truthful autobiographies that I have ever read' – Melvyn Bragg

☐ *The Winning Streak* **Goldsmith and Clutterbuck**   £2.95

Marks & Spencer, Saatchi & Saatchi, United Biscuits, GEC . . . The UK's top companies reveal their formulas for success, in an important and stimulating book that no British manager can afford to ignore.

☐ *The First World War* **A. J. P. Taylor**   £4.95

'He manages in some 200 illustrated pages to say almost everything that is important . . . A special text . . . a remarkable collection of photographs' – *Observer*

PENGUINS ON HEALTH, SPORT AND KEEPING FIT

☐ *Medicines* Peter Parish   £4.95

Fifth Edition. The usages, dosages and adverse effects of all medicines obtainable on prescription or over the counter are covered in this reference guide, designed for the ordinary reader and everyone in health care.

☐ *Baby & Child* Penelope Leach   £7.95

A fully illustrated, expert and comprehensive handbook on the first five years of life. 'It stands head and shoulders above anything else available at the moment' – Mary Kenny in the *Spectator*

☐ *Vogue Natural Health and Beauty*
Bronwen Meredith   £7.50

Health foods, yoga, spas, recipes, natural remedies and beauty preparations are all included in this superb, fully illustrated guide and companion to the bestselling *Vogue Body and Beauty Book*.

☐ *Pregnancy and Diet* Rachel Holme   £1.95

With suggested foods, a sample diet-plan of menus and advice on nutrition, this guide shows you how to avoid excessive calories but still eat well and healthily during pregnancy.

☐ *The Penguin Bicycle Handbook* Rob van der Plas   £4.95

Choosing a bicycle, maintenance, accessories, basic tools, safety, keeping fit – all these subjects and more are covered in this popular, fully illustrated guide to the total bicycle lifestyle.

☐ *Physical Fitness*   £1.25

Containing the 5BX 11-minute-a-day plan for men and the XBX 12-minute-a-day plan for women, this book illustrates the famous programmes originally developed by the Royal Canadian Air Force and now used successfully all over the world.

PENGUINS ON HEALTH,
SPORT AND KEEPING FIT

□ **Audrey Eyton's F-Plus** £1.95

F-Plan menus for women who lunch at work * snack eaters * keen cooks * freezer-owners * busy dieters using convenience foods * overweight children * drinkers and non-drinkers. 'Your short-cut to the most sensational diet of the century' – *Daily Express*

□ **The F-Plan Calorie Counter and Fibre Chart**
Audrey Eyton £1.95

An indispensable companion to the F-Plan diet. High-fibre fresh, canned and packaged foods are listed, there's a separate chart for drinks, *plus* a wonderful selection of effortless F-Plan meals.

□ **The Parents A–Z** Penelope Leach £6.95

From the expert author of *Baby & Child*, this skilled, intelligent and comprehensive guide is by far the best reference book currently available for parents, whether your children are six months, six or sixteen years.

□ **Woman's Experience of Sex** Sheila Kitzinger £5.95

Fully illustrated with photographs and line drawings, this book explores the riches of women's sexuality at every stage of life. 'A book which any mother could confidently pass on to her daughter – and her partner too' – *Sunday Times*

□ **Alternative Medicine** Andrew Stanway £3.25

From Acupuncture and Alexander Technique to Macrobiotics and Yoga, Dr Stanway provides an informed and objective guide to thirty-two therapies in alternative medicine.

□ **Pregnancy** Dr Jonathan Scher and Carol Dix £2.95

Containing the most up-to-date information on pregnancy – the effects of stress, sexual intercourse, drugs, diet, late maternity and genetic disorders – this book is an invaluable and reassuring guide for prospective parents.

PENGUINS ON HEALTH, SPORT AND KEEPING FIT

☐ *Jane Fonda's Workout Book*   £6.95

Help yourself to better looks, superb fitness and a whole new approach to health and beauty with Jane Fonda's world famous programme of exercise and diet advice. Fully illustrated.

☐ *Our Bodies Ourselves* **British edition by
Angela Phillips and Jill Rakusen**   £7.95

Described by the *Guardian* as 'The Bible of the women's health movement', this is the most successful book about women's health ever published, and it has already sold over one million copies worldwide.

These books should be available at all good bookshops or news-agents, but if you live in the UK or the Republic of Ireland and have difficulty in getting to a bookshop, they can be ordered by post. Please indicate the titles required and fill in the form below.

NAME _____ BLOCK CAPITALS

ADDRESS _____

_____

_____

Enclose a cheque or postal order payable to The Penguin Bookshop to cover the total price of books ordered, plus 50p for postage. Readers in the Republic of Ireland should send £1R equivalent to the sterling prices, plus 67p for postage. Send to: The Penguin Book-shop, 54/56 Bridlesmith Gate, Nottingham, NG1 2GP.

You can also order by phoning (0602) 599295, and quoting your Barclaycard or Access number.

Every effort is made to ensure the accuracy of the price and availability of books at the time of going to press, but it is sometimes necessary to increase prices and in these circumstances retail prices may be shown on the covers of books which may differ from the prices shown in this list or elsewhere. This list is not an offer to supply any book.

This order service is only available to residents in the UK and the Republic of Ireland.